Michael van Straten

super health

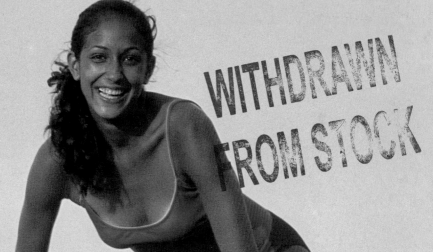

detox

quadrille

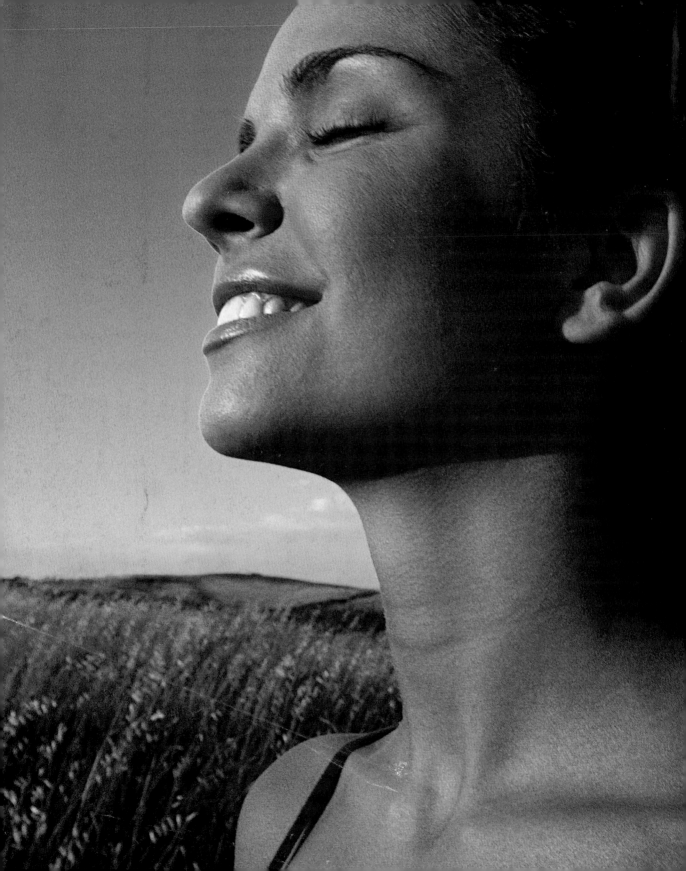

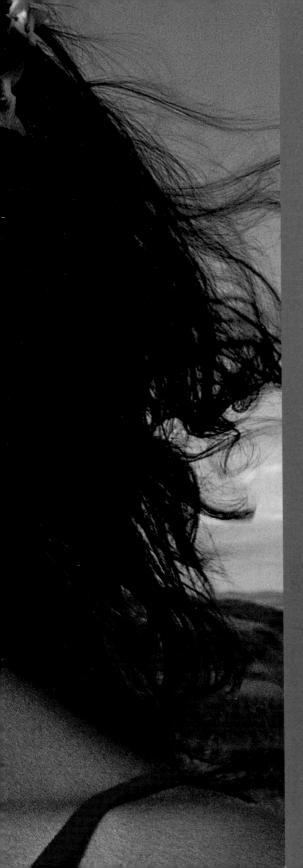

contents

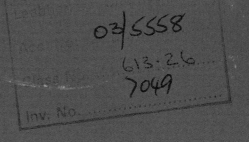

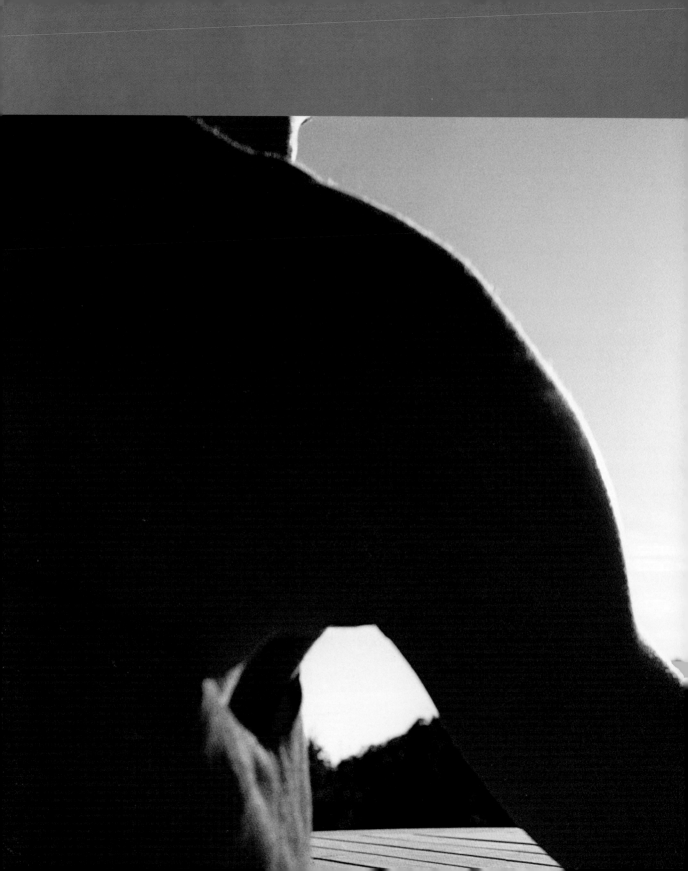

part 1 the detox programmes

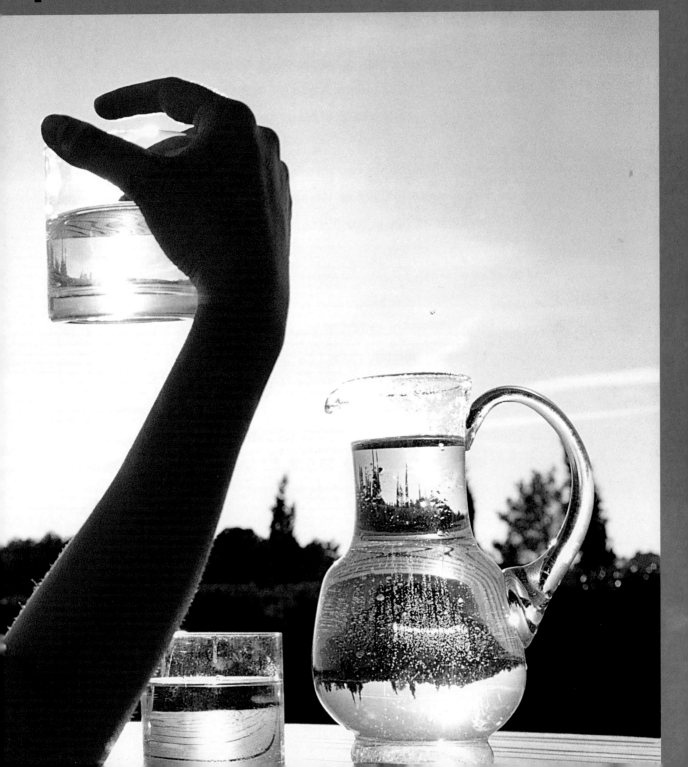

the search for super health

Many factors affect your health but there are only two over which you have no control whatsoever. You can't choose your parents, so you're stuck with whatever genetic influences they pass on. Nor can you plan for acts of God. That said, the vast majority of other health problems you're likely to have are, to a greater or lesser extent, in your own hands.

Can it possibly be that simple? Amazingly, the answer is, yes it can. And detoxing for health is the foundation you need in order to build up strength, resilience, resistance to infection, immunity to the polluted world we live in and a long, productive and enjoyable life.

After 40 years in practice as a naturopath, osteopath and acupuncturist, there is almost nothing that people do regarding their health that surprises me any more. But I am still constantly amazed at the way in which people take up the most extreme attitudes and practices when it comes to health-related issues.

On the one hand, there is a sizable proportion of people who never give a second thought to what they eat or drink, how they live their lives, or what detrimental impact their lifestyles can have on both their minds and their bodies. They totally ignore even the most sensible of health warnings. They simply don't care or can't be bothered.

At the oppposite end of the scale are those who adopt, hook, line and sinker, every extreme health idea that's ever promoted in our 'soundbite', headline-grabbing media. These are the health fanatics, the small minority who follow the most draconian of regimes in pursuit of the holy grail of thinness and eternal youth. It's this group of extremists that worries me most, as they are far more likely to suffer long-term health damage than those with a relaxed attitude to diet and lifestyle. These health fanatics, mostly young women, are easy prey for every new, high-profile health guru who turns up in the media. They end up on diets that fail to supply the most basic nutritional needs, they frequently over-exercise and they are nearly always too thin. In addition, they subject themselves to ridiculous therapies, bogus allergy tests and questionable, if not frankly dangerous, practices like colonic irrigation. As a result, they run the risk of developing a host of health problems ranging from eating disorders to osteoporosis.

What makes this scenario even more worrying is when these extremists apply their latest health craze to their children and decide to bring them up on unrealistic, very restricted and highly dangerous diets.

This is not the way to super health but an almost certain way to a life of ill health and unhappiness. The pressure that these extreme regimes puts upon friends, families and partners is a major factor, too. Normal social life becomes impossible, the pleasure of an enjoyable meal at a convivial table is lost forever and an insupportable strain is placed on any normal relationship.

There are great dangers to the health of our society in the way many people live, but you can minimize these risks for yourself with a little bit of self-discipline, some very modest lifestyle changes, and the inclusion of a wider selection of the most delicious foods. So dump any forms of extremism. That's not the way to super health. Instead, just follow my simple Super Health Detox plan and give your body the tools it needs to maintain a long, happy and disease-free life.

beating the odds

In spite of the extraordinary advances in modern medicine, the health and survival odds are stacked against you. Life expectancy is longer than ever but morbidity is getting worse. Yes, it is true that many illnesses are diseases of old age and as we live longer we are more at risk of developing a host of health problems. But what about the diseases of our modern civilization? Although in the western world better drains, cleaner water and improved hygiene have put an end to mass epidemics of typhoid, dysentery and cholera, these have been replaced with other scourges – high blood pressure, strokes, raised cholesterol, heart disease, late-onset diabetes, cancer, asthma, obesity, gallstones, inflammatory bowel disease, irritable bowel syndrome, PMS, osteoporosis, menopause problems, headaches and even migraine.

One of the reasons is that, as well as eating food that fails to provide our bodies with the optimum amount of protective nutrients, we also live in a world that is increasingly polluted and toxic. Following the occasional detox plan without making long-term changes to your lifestyle and eating habits is only papering over the cracks. But using Super Health Detox will help you on both counts.

For example, the toxic chemicals in many household products can affect your immune system, reducing its effectiveness and paving the way for ill health. And when your children are exposed to these chemicals, you put their health at risk too, regardless of how well you may be feeding them. And these are risks that can stay with them for life.

in the kitchen

The words kitchen and hygiene go together like bread and jam, but many common cleaning products are highly toxic and food containers, plastic film or your brand new vinyl flooring may be just as bad.

washing-up liquids

Most contain synthetic musk fragrances which are persistent and toxic chemicals. Residues can be left on cutlery and crockery that is not well rinsed, and these residues will then contaminate food. They can also be absorbed through the skin and because they dissolve in fat, they end up as long-term deposits in the body, posing a threat to all of us but especially to small children. Look out for 'green' versions and the better supermarket own-label products. The good ones will list all the ingredients, but the risky ones won't.

anti-bacterial surface cleaners

These too contain hazardous synthetic musks, but consumers are brainwashed to believe these cleaners are necessary to kill every known bug. However, there is growing evidence that this obsession with over-zealous hygiene is one probable cause of the ever-increasing amount of childhood allergies. So when you need to disinfect a surface, buy one of the environmentally safer products or save your money and use vinegar and hot water.

oven cleaners

These are likely to contain highly toxic chemicals called phthalates (see Plastics, below) as well as synthetic musks. 'Green' versions are available, but they may need a bit more elbow-grease.

fabric softeners and laundry products

Yet more products containing synthetic musks – now so widespread that they can be found in almost everyone's body fat – and women accumulate twice as much as men. They even turn up in breast milk so are a serious danger to your baby. 'Green' alternatives are widely available.

plastics

Plastics are a major hazard to babies and small children. Vinyl flooring is made from PVC and to keep it pliable, it contains chemicals called phthalates. These plasticizers have serious, damaging effects because they interfere with our hormones and have been blamed for early puberty, birth defects, damage to testicles and infertility. Some plasticizers have already been banned from the plastics used in teething rings and soft toys for small children. But they're still in your vinyl floor tiles and from here they are released into the atmosphere.

Replace vinyl with linoleum which is non-toxic and has natural antiseptic properties. Slate, quarry tiles or natural wood are also ideal alternatives, as is natural cork flooring. It's warmer and 100 per cent non-toxic.

Polystyrene food containers are also made with chemicals that are believed to affect human oestrogens. To prevent toxic substances getting into food, avoid direct contact with plastic film by keeping food in glass or ceramic containers with the film stretched over the top.

down the toilet, in the air

Most toilet descalers contain synthetic musks as do air fresheners. The most dangerous of these is xylene, which is known to cause cancer in animals. Lavatory bleaches are one of the worst culprits. Apart from being extremely poisonous, nearly all contain highly toxic chlorine. This converts to organochlorines which persist in the environment and are stored in body tissues. As a safe and environmentally friendly alternative, use baking soda or white vinegar, left in the toilet overnight.

on your skin

When you're out shopping for soap, stick to the natural, eco-friendly sort. They're better for your skin too.

lurking in the carpet

You may be surprised to learn that your carpet could well contain adhesives which release volatile organic compounds (VOCs) into the air. It also probably plays host to a wealth of chemicals that are designed to resist stains, repel moths, kill dustmites or prevent static. These are all potentially damaging to humans but worryingly, some samples taken from carpets have also been found to contain tributyl tin (TBT). This is one of the most potent endocrine-disrupting chemicals there is and is a definite cause of sexual mutation in animals.

On top of this, insecticides, pesticides, solvents, air fresheners, lead, mercury, dustmite droppings and a host of other damaging substances are found in carpet dust. These can affect both children and adults and are among the causes of ever-increasing asthma. Wooden flooring is a wonderful alternative but avoid laminates as these use toxic adhesives. Sisal, coir and seagrass are all good alternatives and are mostly grown without the use of chemicals.

furniture polish

Before using polish, take care, as most manufacturers will not disclose the chemicals they use and I can only assume they must be nasty, otherwise they'd come clean. Traditional beeswax may be harder work, but it won't release VOCs into the air at home for your family to inhale.

insecticides

Avoid anti-dustmite insecticides, especially in a child's room. They are a permanent risk and can be inhaled or get onto the skin.

smoke

The autumn garden bonfire may give off frightening amounts of poisonous smoke, as may the cosy wood fire in your grate.

lead

This is one of the most dangerous substances, especially because it is has a cumulative effect. Modern paints are not allowed to contain lead so it's mainly the old lead-based paints that are the cause of concern. If you live in an old house, get professional advice before redecorating. Never rub down old lead-based paint or use a blowtorch on it, nor burn old windows, doors or other painted timber. And watch out for the fact that many older houses may still contain sections of lead piping in their water system. If you're worried, contact your water supplier.

solvents

Paints, stains, varnishes and wood preservatives – even some water-based versions – also contain solvents, which can be just as worrying as lead. These solvents can affect blood cells, and may trigger asthma, headaches and migraine. And like all volatile organic compounds (VOCs), they contribute to summer smog. There are lots of natural alternatives to choose from on the market.

outdoors

If there's one place that must be organic, it should be your own garden. Garden chemicals are highly damaging to the immune system and are a common cause of accidental poisoning in children. Many natural alternatives are now available. Remember, too, that exterior timber is mostly treated with arsenic compounds which leach into soil leaving a highly toxic residue. This residue gets into grass and plants, and is brought into the house on human and animal feet, adding to the toxic chemical load deposited forever in your flooring. Again, there are alternative timber treatments, so ask before buying fencing, decking and play equipment.

time to detox?

Everyone, no matter how super-healthy they may be, would benefit from the occasional detox. But some people's need is more serious. To find out how much you need Super Health Detox, answer these questions – truthfully as the only person you'll be cheating is yourself – then work out your score.

1 How many times a week do you eat breakfast?
- **A** Every day.
- **B** Most days if I've got time.
- **C** Breakfast? Does coffee and biscuits at 11 o'clock count?

2 You know you should be eating five portions of fruit and vegetables a day. What does that consist of?
- **A** Apples, oranges, bananas, greens, salads – any I can lay my hands on.
- **B** Will five grapes and a portion of chips do?
- **C** Who says I have to eat five pieces of fruit a day? I hate the stuff.

3 How much of the food you eat consists of processed food like burgers, sausages and frozen TV dinners?
- **A** None – I like cooking proper meals.
- **B** Not much – but I do eat them three or four times a week when I'm busy.
- **C** Most of it – I don't have time to cook.

4 When you use oil or fat for cooking, what type is it?
- **A** Good olive oil.
- **B** Sunflower or other seed oil.
- **C** Butter, lard or hard margarine.

5 How often do you eat oily fish like sardines, salmon and mackerel?
- **A** At least once a week – I know it's good for me.

- **B** Probably not that often, but I know I should eat more.
- **C** I don't think they sell them at our chippie.

6 What type of milk do you normally buy?
- **A** Mostly skimmed – I'm watching my weight.
- **B** Semi-skimmed – it doesn't taste as good as ordinary milk but I know it's healthier.
- **C** Full fat – the others are all revolting.

7 Bread is the staff of life. Which do you normally choose?
- **A** Wholemeal – the fibre keeps me regular.
- **B** A variety, I like all sorts.
- **C** I never touch bread, it's fattening.

8 Do you (tick as many as you like)
 Smoke?
 Drink more than 14 units (women) or 21 units (men) of alcohol a week?
 Take sleeping pills/tranquillisers/antidepressants?
 Use recreational drugs?

9 Which of the following sums up your exercise pattern?
- **A** I exercise loads – I practically live at the gym.
- **B** I don't do as much as I should, but I do play tennis/football or kick a ball around with the kids three or four times a week.
- **C** Well, I walk from the bus/car to the supermarket/pub door.

10 How often do you make time to do something you want?

    A At least once a week – I know I need to spoil myself occasionally.

    B Not that often, but I probably get a break once a month or so.

    C Never – my job/the kids/the home are far too demanding.

11 Have you ever suffered from constipation?

    A No.

    B From time to time, but it has never been a serious problem.

    C I've had it for as long as I can remember.

12 The lift's broken and you walk up three floors, or you make a dash for the bus. How breathless are you?

    A Not at all.

    B A little, but it only lasts a couple of minutes.

    C I think I'm dying and it takes 10 minutes to get my breath back.

13 How many times a year do you catch a cold or flu?

    A Hardly ever.

    B Two or three.

    C I've lost count – if there's a bug around I get it.

14 How often do you get headaches (apart from migraine) and have to take painkillers?

    A Once in a blue moon.

    B Occasionally.

    C Most days.

15 In the last twelve months, how many courses of antibiotics have you been prescribed by your doctor?

    A 2 or less.

    B 3–5

    C I've lost count.

Score:
A – 1 point
B – 3 points
C or tick – 5 points

Over 85 – start detoxing now and check your life insurance policy. This is not the time to buy **War and Peace** – you may not be around long enough to finish reading it!

60–85 – all is not lost. A few changes to your eating and lifestyle, a bit more exercise and you'll soon be in better health. Pay special attention to the rebuilding for health regime (see pages 38–41).

35–60 – you're doing a great job. You're probably eating well, taking some exercise, have a good understanding about how your body works, but still having fun.

under 35 – you win the booby prize! You may be super healthy but your life is very dull. You're probably a food freak and a hypochondriac, worrying about everything you put in your mouth and the health risks of everything that's pleasurable in life. Lighten up and remember that in the concert of life there is no rehearsal. You might be a health fanatic but you could be struck by lightning tomorrow.

I'm sure you've worked it out by now, but all the As are the healthiest or correct answers, Bs not quite right, Cs and ticks mean bad news.

cleansing for

Cleanliness is next to godliness so most people wash, bathe or shower every day, but how often do you think about cleansing the inside? Apart from the toxic chemicals you absorb from the environment and from your food and drink, the body also produces its own waste. Much of this is eliminated naturally, but some remains in the body as unwanted chemical by-products and free radicals and these will all eventually harm your health. Fasting is a way of getting rid of them. It will also increase your blood's white-cell count which will help boost your natural immunity and protect you from disease.

when should I detox?

As a naturopath I strongly advise the regular – ideally once a week – use of a twenty-four hour juice and water fast as a way of maintaining good health. If regular twenty-four hour fasting doesn't appeal to you, then a forty-eight hour regime, not more than once a month, is an extremely effective health-inducing body cleanser. I offer a structured forty-eight hour programme, but if you want, you could go for two days on just water and juices. If you do this though, by the end of the second day you'll feel a certain amount of light-headedness, so it's advisable not to undertake strenuous physical activity, drive or use dangerous machinery.

For a seasonal clear-out, a three-day regime is ideal. It's also a great way to help your body recover from illness, but seek medical advice before starting if you've recently been ill. The three-day programme consists largely of a combination of water, juices, clear soups and some fresh fruit and vegetables. This fast is not suitable while you're working and should be fitted in when you can have at least one day to recover. For example, you could start at work on Friday, complete the fast on Saturday and Sunday, then have Monday as a day off.

health

side effects

The most common side effect of fasting is headache. This is caused partly by the drop in blood-sugar levels and the beginnings of elimination, but often it's caused by the body being deprived of caffeine. The more coffee you usually drink, the worse the headache is likely to be. Don't resort to painkillers; simply drink lots more water and it will pass.

During forty-eight hour or three-day fasts you may also get what naturopaths call a 'healing crisis' – a coated tongue, bad breath, increased temperature, sweating, tremors and general aches and pains. This is traditionally believed to be caused by the sudden release of accumulated toxins from the body. We now know that it's the result of the natural bacteria in the gut dying off and releasing chemicals which are then absorbed by the gut wall. Don't worry if any of these things happen to you; they're a good sign.

take care

As I've already said, if you've recently been ill you should check with your doctor before starting any fast. Similarly, if you have an underlying illness like diabetes or you are on prescribed medication that needs to be taken with food – non-steroidal anti-inflammatories for example – you especially need to exercise caution and consult your regular physician. Take care if you suffer from migraine, as fasting can trigger attacks and, although short detox periods are fine during pregnancy and breastfeeding, you should not go longer than one day.

And to do the best you can for your body, during your detox try and consume only organic produce and, if possible, make your own juices. Now's the time to invest in that juicer!

the extras

Detoxing is not simply giving up food. You need to take care about what and how much you drink and about how much exercise you need. In addition, my experience has shown that taking some commonly available food supplements while you detox will ensure your body benefits to the maximum.

what to drink

First thing in the morning make up a jug of Parsley Tea (see recipe, page 83), keep it in the fridge and drink small glasses regularly throughout the day. This gentle diuretic will help to speed up the detoxifying and cleansing processes, so make sure you drink it all.

You can drink as much water, herb or weak China tea as you like, but don't add milk or any form of sweetening. And you must not consume fizzy water, canned drinks, squashes, cordials, alcohol, Indian tea, coffee or any sweetened drinks. This includes sugar-free commercial products which contain artificial sweeteners.

the supplements

No matter whether you choose to do a twenty-four hour cleansing detox, or the forty-eight hour or three-day versions, you can improve the efficiency of the programme and support your body's whole system by taking the appropriate supplements every day.

for general well-being

During all these programmes you will be consuming far less food than normal and even though the recommended foods will provide an abundance of nutrients, it is important to give the body an extra supportive boost of vitamins and minerals to avoid any possible deficiencies and to guarantee optimum levels. For this reason you should take:

▶ 1 high-potency multi-vitamin and mineral supplement (choose one of the reputable brand leaders)
▶ 500mg vitamin C, three times a day. If you can find it, use ester-C which many leading manufacturers now include in their products as it is non-acidic and less likely to cause digestive upsets – especially important while you're eating less food

• A one-a-day standardized extract of cynarin – from globe artichokes. This stimulates liver function and helps the body eliminate fat-soluble substances stored in the liver.

for bowel function

Maintaining proper and regular bowel function is especially important during a detox as you will have a much lower fibre intake than normal.

• To stimulate, improve and maintain bowel function take 1–2 tablespoons of oat bran or ground psyllium seed every night while you follow the plan, and for best results start the day with a glass of hot water with the juice of a lemon, described as a tonic rather than you have.

for a weak immune system

If your immune system has obviously been under par, then detoxing will help boost your immune function, and you may also particularly take these nutritional supplements:

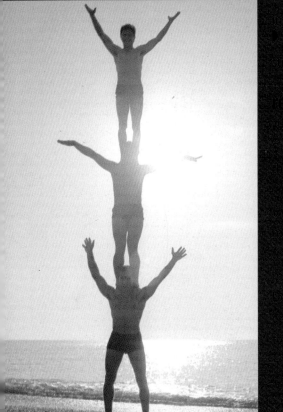

rest and exercise

twenty-four hour cleansing

If you've had a week of entertaining clients, business lunches and over-indulgence, or have been to a couple of great parties and had a bit too much alcohol, this twenty-four hour Cleansing for Health fast will flush out your system and revitalise your mind and body. Even if you're not suffering from any self-inflicted damage, it's an excellent way of compensating for the unavoidable environmental hazards we're constantly exposed to and will give you a short, sharp, good-health boost.

This twenty-four hour detox can easily be incorporated into even the most hectic of lifestyles. Though best done on a non-working day, most people in reasonably good health can manage the fast even while working. Used on a regular, weekly, basis, it represents a huge investment in your good health.

on waking	A large glass of hot water with a thick slice of organic unwaxed lemon
breakfast	A large glass of hot water with a thick slice of organic unwaxed lemon A mug of Ginger Tea (see recipe, page 83)
mid-morning	A large glass of hot water with a thick slice of organic unwaxed lemon
lunch	A large glass of Tomato Juice and Celery Blend (see recipe, page 82) A mug of Ginger Tea (see recipe, page 83)
mid-afternoon	A large glass of hot water with a thick slice of organic unwaxed lemon
supper	Kiwi and Pineapple Juice (see recipe, page 82) A mug of Ginger Tea (see recipe, page 83)
evening	Orange Juice and Almond Blend (see recipe, page 82)
bedtime	A mug of camomile tea (any reputable brand) with a teaspoon of organic honey

forty-eight hour cleansing

If a one-day-a-week detox doesn't appeal to you, you might prefer a forty-eight hour regime that you do once a month. Start by following the twenty-four hour Cleansing for Health fast, then for the next twenty-four hours have:

on waking   A large glass of hot water with a thick slice of organic unwaxed lemon

breakfast   A large glass of hot water with a thick slice of organic unwaxed lemon
An orange
Half a pink grapefruit
A slice of cantaloupe melon
A mug of camomile tea

mid-morning   A large glass of hot water with a thick slice of organic unwaxed lemon

lunch   A large plate of mixed raw red and yellow pepper, cucumber, carrot, radishes, tomatoes, celery and broccoli, with a handful of chopped fresh parsley and a drizzle of extra-virgin olive oil and lemon juice
A large glass of apple juice
A mug of mint tea

mid-afternoon   A large glass of hot water with a thick slice of organic unwaxed lemon

supper   A large bowl of fresh fruit salad, to include apple, pear, grapes, mango and some berries – but no banana
A handful of raisins – make sure to chew them very slowly – and a handful of fresh, unsalted cashew nuts
A glass of unsalted mixed vegetable juice (any reputable brand)

evening   A large glass of hot water with a thick slice of organic unwaxed lemon

bedtime   A mug of camomile tea with a teaspoon of organic honey

three-day cleansing

A three-day detox is quite a serious undertaking. Though not strictly speaking a fast, other than on the first day, you will feel noticeable side effects so this programme is definitely best done when you are not working. Because of your very low calorie intake, you will certainly feel quite light-headed by the end of day two and even more so during day three. Any severe headaches will pass and towards the end, you may begin to feel euphoric.

Because this is a cleansing regime, as your body steps up its eliminating processes, it's likely that you will develop unpleasant breath, a coated tongue and will pass urine more frequently than normal. It's essential that you keep your fluid intake up to the recommended level to replace any fluid you have lost and to stimulate further elimination. It's unlikely that you will have any unusual problems with wind, but even though you're eating much less bulk than normal, you may find that your bowels are more active, especially in the latter part of day three.

Take care when you return to normal eating after this three-day plan. I recommend you follow the eight-day return to normal eating programme, but if you don't have time for that, just make sure you don't overload your digestive system. Eat little and often, avoid all animal protein, all high-fat and fried foods, and apart from yoghurt, avoid all other dairy products. On day four you will need to drink at least one and a half litres of fluid. You can eat any fruit and vegetables and introduce some starchy food in the form of oats, wholemeal bread, rice and pasta. A small amount of grilled, poached or steamed white fish would be fine, but don't have shellfish, seafood or oily fish.

Days 1 and 2, follow the Forty-Eight Hour Cleansing programme. Day 3:

on waking A large glass of hot water with a thick slice of organic unwaxed lemon.

breakfast A large glass of hot water with a thick slice of organic unwaxed lemon.
A carton of organic low-fat live yoghurt with a teaspoon of honey, a dessertspoon of raisins and a dessertspoon of chopped hazelnuts.
A glass of half-orange, half-grapefruit juice.

mid-morning A large glass of Carrot, Apple and Celery Juice (see recipe, page 83).
4 dried apricots
4 prunes

lunch A large glass of hot water with a thick slice of organic unwaxed lemon.
Carrot and Red Cabbage Salad (see recipe, page 108).
A mug of mint tea.

mid-afternoon A glass of any unsweetened fruit juice.

supper A mixture of chopped steamed leek, cabbage, spinach and kale, drizzled with olive oil, lemon juice and a generous sprinkling of nutmeg.
A glass of unsweetened red grape juice.
A mug of lime blossom tea.

evening 4 prunes
4 dates
A small bunch of black grapes.

bedtime A cup of China tea with two rice crackers.

eight-day return to normal eating

If you've managed to do the full three-day detox, you're obviously serious about getting your health back on target. Now follow this eight-day plan to reaccustom your body to normal eating and maximize the health benefits. The plan provides large quantities of protective and health-promoting antioxidants, which are good for your heart, circulation, blood pressure and cholesterol. They also give your body a valuable cancer-protective boost, while at the same time providing an abundance of the essential basic nutrients.

If you've only done the twenty-four hour programme, then this plan is pretty much optional, but I do suggest you try to follow it for just two days. If you've done the forty-eight hour programme, then you should follow at least the first two days of the plan.

It's extremely important that you follow day 1 exactly as it's laid out, but the following seven days are more flexible and within each day you may switch light meals and main meals to suit your lifestyle. You can also switch whole days around, but don't mix meals from one day with meals from another as this upsets the balance of the eating plan.

keeping up your fluid intake

While you're doing this, you must keep your fluid intake up to a minimum of one and a half litres a day, but the same rules about canned drinks and commercial juices apply as for the detox programmes. Many people find that once they've got into the habit of starting each day with hot water and lemon, it becomes a valuable addition to their normal regime. It avoids the early morning caffeine shot, stimulates the digestive system and helps to get your bowels moving regularly.

And now you've managed to reduce your caffeine intake, try to keep it down. There's nothing wrong with two or three cups a day of your favourite tea or good coffee, but more than this is not a long-term health benefit as excessive amounts of caffeine can be a factor in raising your blood pressure.

day 1

on waking   A large glass of hot water with a thick slice of organic unwaxed lemon

breakfast   A helping of fresh-fruit salad consisting of apple, pear, grapes, mango and pineapple with
a carton of low-fat live yoghurt and a tablespoon of good quality unsweetened muesli
A mug of any herb tea

mid-morning   6 dried apricots
A glass of unsweetened pineapple juice

lunch   A large bowl of Lettuce Soup (see recipe, page 99) with a chunk of My Easy Bread (see
recipe, page 78) – no butter
A cup of any herb or China tea

mid-afternoon   1 apple
1 pear

supper   Pasta with Lettuce Pesto (see recipe, page 85)
A cup of any herb or China tea

day 2

on waking   A large glass of hot water with a thick slice of organic unwaxed lemon

breakfast   Half a pink grapefruit
Poached Eggs and Tomatoes (see recipe, page 79)

light meal   1 avocado and 2 large spoons of cottage cheese
Large bunch of grapes

main meal   Cucumber and Strawberry Salad (see recipe, page 103)
Mixed Vegetable Stir-fry with Rice (see recipe, page 84)

day 3

breakfast   One large peach with any seasonal berries

light meal   Large green salad of watercress, celery, raw spinach, basil, coriander, chicory and dark lettuce like cos, with a portion of steamed carrots, courgettes, peas, broad beans and sweetcorn, tossed in a mean teaspoon of butter, sprinkled with chopped mint.

main meal   A bowl of Vegetable Soup (see recipe, page 99)
A large Stuffed Red Pepper (see recipe, page 96)
Two pieces of fresh fruit – not bananas

day 4

breakfast   A large bowl of cherries or other seasonal berries with a carton of plain, low-fat live yoghurt

light meal   Mixed green salad
Pasta all'Aglio e Olio (see recipe, page 89)

main meal   Tsatsiki (see recipe, page 104)
Grilled Chicken Breast on Iceberg Lettuce (see recipe, page 85) with grilled tomato and baby new potatoes boiled in their skins
A large peach

day 5

breakfast   Porridge Muesli (see recipe, page 78)
A banana

light meal   A wholemeal pitta bread filled with sliced hardboiled egg, chopped tomato, cucumber, raw fennel and shredded lettuce

main meal   Celery Salad (see recipe, page 104)
Baked Stuffed Trout (see recipe, page 87) served with warm runner beans tossed in a drizzle of olive oil and a squeeze of lemon juice and sprinkled with chopped spring onions and parsley

day 6

breakfast   A large bunch of grapes

light meal   A bowl of Vegetable Soup (see recipe, page 99) with a wholemeal roll
A selection of washed, sliced raw vegetables to include radishes, carrot, fennel, celery and olives
A ripe pear

main meal   Veggie Curry with Rice (see recipe, page 87)
Tomato, Red Onion and Beetroot Salad (see recipe, page 105)
Two kiwi fruit

day 7

breakfast   A selection of mixed succulent fruits such as strawberries, raspberries, currants, apricots and peach

light meal   Tuna and Cottage-Cheese Stuffed Tomato (see recipe, page 88) with a small green salad and two slices of My Easy Bread (see recipe, page 78)

main meal   Stir-Fried Tofu with Vegetables and Noodles (see recipe, page 88)
A glass of Berry Smoothie (see recipe, page 83)

day 8

breakfast   Two organic free-range boiled eggs with one slice of wholemeal toast and butter
A large glass of freshly squeezed orange juice

light meal   Mushrooms with Radicchio and Chicory (see recipe, page 85) with 1 slice of wholemeal bread
An apple and a pear

main meal   Grapefruit, Peach and Fromage Frais Salad (see recipe, page 105)
Grilled Salmon Steak (see recipe, page 89) served with boiled potatoes and any green vegetable you fancy
A matchbox-sized (not the giant-sized cook's matches!) piece of your favourite cheese with a stick of celery, a handful of radishes and two rye crispbreads

cleansing summary

Well done! It's not always as easy as it looks but having completed the Cleansing for Health programme, you certainly deserve a pat on the back. But your reward is much greater than that. If you have carefully followed the programme right through, this is where you'll be.

what you've achieved

▶ You'll have helped your body eliminate a lot of toxic residues

▶ You'll have cleansed your urinary system with a massive increase of fluid throughput, so reducing your chances of urinary infection

▶ You'll have rested your liver by drastically reducing the amount of fat in your diet and by avoiding the enormous number of chemical flavourings, colourings, preservatives and additives used in most commercially prepared foods

▶ You'll have given your entire digestive system a healthy holiday by cutting out most animal protein and greatly increasing your consumption of fruit and vegetables

▶ You'll certainly have shortened the time it takes for food to pass through your digestive system and short food-transit times are a major factor in reducing the risk of inflammatory bowel disease and bowel cancer.

how you feel

If you've got to the end of any of the programmes successfully the benefits will be glaringly obvious:

▶ You'll feel pleased with yourself for completing a difficult task. The good news is that it will be much easier next time

▶ You'll feel lighter in spirit as detoxing sharpens the mind and improves focus and concentration. It's not a coincidence that both ancient and modern mystics and religious teachers used fasting as a way of increasing their spiritual awareness and their ability to focus on solving great problems

▶ You'll feel lighter in body and you'll certainly have lost some weight if you needed to, but this lightness is not just because you're carrying a smaller physical load. It's because your whole metabolic process will be running at its most efficient and will now be firing on all cylinders

▶ You'll feel more healthy as your metabolism expends less energy on wasteful tasks like dealing with junk food and excessive alcohol and is able instead to concentrate on converting what you eat into readily available energy.

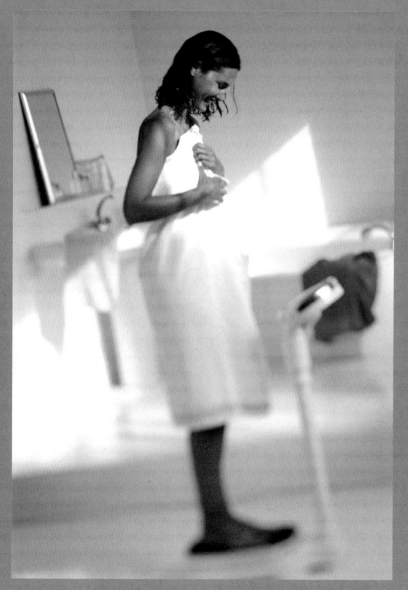

But if you didn't achieve your goals, what you certainly mustn't do is feel guilty. It's also important not to give up on the whole programme just because you were tempted and fell by the wayside on day 5. Just go back to the day before you fell from grace, and start again. You'll still reap the rewards.

replenishing

You're doing well and your health is on the up and up. You've detoxed and cleansed and now it's time to look to the longer term. Even if you haven't spent the last five years living on junk food and burning the candle at both ends, you probably haven't followed the most healthy of eating patterns. You've looked at some of the cranky health and diet books and thought, quite rightly, that living on a vegan or macrobiotic diet, going to your friends for dinner with a brown paper bag full of mung beans, grated carrot and a bottle of your own freshly made wheatgrass juice is not quite your cup of tea. So what else can you do?

the french paradox

You're now going to start replenishing your body's depleted stores of many of the essential nutrients. But you can put away the hair shirt and take a leaf out of pretty well any French or Mediterranean cookbook.

In the early 1990s a French researcher spotted the surprising fact that although his countrymen (and women and children) ate mountains of runny cheese, munched their way through kilos of paté and foie gras, drank litres of wine and smoked hundreds of their unique cigarettes, they suffered 30 per cent less heart disease than people living in northern Europe and the USA. And people in the south of France suffered 30 per cent less than the rest of their compatriots.

Though this phenomenon is now known as the French Paradox, the same sort of results are apparent throughout the Mediterranean countries. What is more, recent studies have shown that men who had already suffered a heart attack and then switched to a Mediterranean diet cut their chances of a second attack by 70 per cent. Not surprisingly this news has made the French Paradox even more exciting.

for health

Naturopaths like me have been advocating French and Mediterranean styles of eating for a hundred years. Prevention of heart disease is just one benefit. Less bowel cancer, fewer circulatory problems, fewer gallstones, less osteoporosis and rheumatic disease are some others. That's because a Mediterranean diet

▶ is lower in saturated fatty acids – the animal fats that are a major contributor to heart disease
▶ is rich in polyunsaturated fatty acids from vegetable oils, which do not cause heart disease
▶ is very rich in mono-unsaturated fatty acids from olive oil, nuts and seeds, which help the body to get rid of cholesterol and protect your heart and arteries
▶ is rich in dietary fibre, which improves digestion and bowel function and protects against some forms of cancer
▶ contains lots of chemicals called polyphenols from red wine, fruits and vegetables, which are protective and anti-ageing antioxidants
▶ consists of less red meat and far more fish and shellfish, which means less bad fat, more good fat and minerals – especially iodine, zinc and selenium – and more Omega-3 fatty acids, which are essential for brain development and are a protective anti-inflammatory
▶ consists of less convenience food, which means a lower fat intake and far less salt.

In a nutshell, to replenish and protect your health long-term, you should enjoy two glasses of red wine every day, at least four portions of vegetables, three of fruit, five to eight servings of good, starchy food like bread, rice, pasta, potatoes or beans, a small portion of meat, fish, poultry, eggs and cheese, and modest quantities of olive, rapeseed or safflower oils.

But don't be a fanatic – a little of what you fancy really does do you good.

seven-day replenishing

Now you come to the replenishing part of the programme. What follows is a week of rainbow eating – lots of brightly coloured fruits, vegetables and salads, all loaded with antioxidants. This is what your body needs to give an enormous boost to its natural protective mechanisms.

This is not a rigid regime. You now have some freedom of choice, but do choose as wide a variety of dishes as possible and don't just stick to the ones you like or which are quicker and easier to prepare. The golden rule though is that you must eat breakfast, one light meal and one main meal every day. This is to ensure that you get a wide spread of the essential vitamins, minerals and trace elements.

the antioxidants

Conventional puddings are off the menu. Instead finish every meal with a generous portion of fresh or cooked fruit. Fruits with the highest antioxidant value are blueberries, blackberries, blackcurrants, redcurrants, cranberries, strawberries, raspberries, cherries, prunes, raisins, dates, figs, dried apricots, kiwi, black grapes, mango, paw paw, passion fruit, citrus fruits, bananas, apples and pears. You need to eat around 500 grams in weight daily of as wide a mixture of these as you can – and that's a minimum. In fact, at least 700 grams in weight of what you eat should consist of fruit, vegetables and salads, and around half your calories should come from the complex carbohydrates – bread, pasta, rice, beans, and so on.

A certain amount of frozen fruit is acceptable as the only serious nutrient loss will be some of the vitamin C, and this is adequately provided elsewhere. But please don't use canned fruits or imagine that the fruits you get in ready-made pies, puddings and desserts will be nearly as good.

If you're a vegetarian, don't overdo the eggs and cheese, and if you're a carnivore you'll be enjoying meat, fish and poultry – but in modest amounts. It's most important to eat three meals a day and you must understand that if you are on any sort of weight loss programme, once your calories drop below 1500 a day, it's difficult to get all the nutrients you need to sustain good health (see pages 54–57).

the anti-nutrients

During this week you need to avoid the anti-nutrients – those foods that sap your health and vitality. So this means no takeaways, burgers, chips, bags of crisps, or high-fat high-sugar cakes, biscuits and pastries. And it's no to instant noodles, soup in a cup, pasties and meat pies – unless you make your own. In fact, you should eat as little ready-made convenience food as you can possibly manage.

added extras

This week will help make good your nutritional deficiencies. Some nutrients, like minerals and the fat-soluble vitamins A, D and E, can be stored by the body, but others need replenishing daily. So continue to take the multivitamin and mineral tablet, as well as the zinc and the probiotic that you were taking during the Cleansing for Health programme and now also take the following daily supplements. Continue with them all through the Rebuilding for Health programme and for at least a month after that.

▶ A one-a-day tablet of selenium with vitamins A, C and E
▶ 500 mg fish oil
▶ A carotenoid supplement which includes lycopene, lutein and betacarotene
▶ BioStrath Elixir – the Swiss herbal medicine that boosts natural immunity. Take 5ml three times a day.

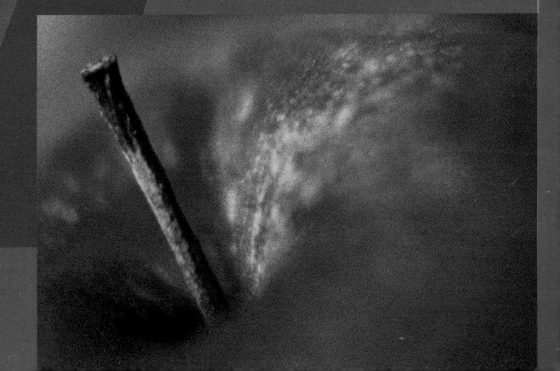

breakfast options

▶ Poached Eggs and Tomatoes (see recipe, page 79) with pink grapefruit juice

▶ Poached Haddock with Cherry Tomatoes (see recipe, page 80) with tomato juice

▶ Kedgeree (see recipe, page 80) with Grape, Pear, Apple and Pineapple Juice (see recipe, page 83)

▶ Dutch Breakfast (see recipe, page 79) with orange juice

▶ Porridge Muesli (see recipe, page 78) with Apple, Kiwi, Pear and Celery Juice (see recipe, page 83)

▶ Any wholewheat cereal with added blueberries, raspberries or strawberries, and sliced banana, and with Kiwi and Pineapple Juice (see recipe, page 82)

▶ Tomato and Mushroom Omelette (see recipe, page 81) with Yoghurt and Prune Smoothie (see recipe, page 83)

light meal options

Three wholemeal bread or pitta pocket sandwiches containing:

▶ A mixture of watercress, grated carrot, cress and chopped, semi-dried apricots mixed with live natural yoghurt, black pepper and a pinch of cayenne; Home-made Chicken Liver Paté (see recipe, page 84) with beansprouts, thinly sliced cucumber and cranberry sauce; or banana sprinkled with lemon juice to stop it going brown, chopped ready-to-eat prunes, dried cranberries and peanut butter

▶ Chicken Soup with Barley (see recipe, page 100)

▶ Borscht (see recipe, page 100)

▶ Thick Bean and Barley Soup (see recipe, page 101)

▶ White Soup (see recipe, page 101)

▶ Fruit Crudités with Ricotta Cheese Dip (see recipe, page 104)

▶ Baked Leeks with Cheese and Eggs (see recipe, page 89)

▶ Falafel (see recipe, page 90)

main meal options

▶ Grilled Chicken Breast on Iceberg Lettuce (see recipe, page 85) with rice and mixed vegetables

▶ Baked Stuffed Trout (see recipe, page 87) with Ratatouille (see recipe, page 86)

▶ Stir-fried Tofu with Vegetables and Noodles (see recipe, page 88)

▶ Pheasant Casserole with Red Cabbage (see recipe, page 90)

▶ Grilled Salmon Steak (see recipe, page 89) with new potatoes, French beans and purple sprouting broccoli

▶ Couscous with Vegetables (see recipe, page 91) with minted yoghurt

▶ Organic Beef Stew with Vegetables (see recipe, page 91) with lots of olive-oil mash (mashed potatoes made with olive oil – no butter, no milk)

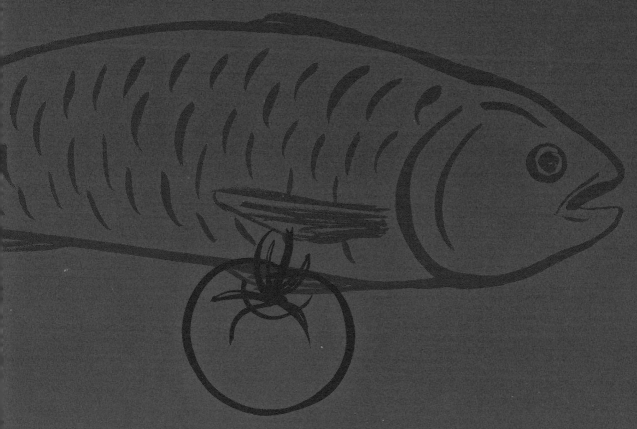

replenishing summary

Once you've followed the detox programmes, including the seven-day replenishing, you'll have given your long-term health an enormous boost and this is what most people are looking to achieve. But the programmes can also be used when short-term intervention is necessary, for example if you're recovering from illness, accident, surgery, or periods of extreme stress, such as bereavement. At times like that, just making the effort to stick to my super-healthy eating plan will occupy your mind and will work as a form of displacement activity. The added bonus is that the excellent nutrition you'll be getting will sustain and support your central nervous system through the battering it's taking. If you've managed to get through the entire programme, these are the benefits you'll be feeling.

what you've achieved

▶ A substantial improvement in your body's reserves of nutrients
▶ Your circulating levels of essential nutrients will have gone up
▶ Your stores of minerals like iron and calcium, selenium and zinc will have increased
▶ Thanks to your increased intake of antioxidants, your immune system will be working harder and the number of T-killer cells in your blood – your main defence against bacteria and viruses – has also increased. This will mean that you're less likely to fall prey to one minor illness after another.

how you feel

You're at an interim stage in your detoxing for health plan and you may feel as though not much is happening. But this is far from the truth. By cleansing and replenishing, you'll have built up a substantial credit in your health deposit account. The impact of the detox is actually immediate, so by now you should be feeling:

▶ More energetic physically

▶ Stronger and more capable of longer periods of exertion

▶ More comfortable and less bloated – your new regular and regulated eating has helped your digestive system no end

▶ More balanced as the regular meals you're now eating are keeping your blood-sugar level on an even keel; the peaks and troughs of frantic activity followed by extreme tiredness are now being ironed out

▶ Happier, because your emotional ups and downs are a thing of the past

▶ Better able to concentrate and with quicker reflexes

▶ That your overall sense of well-being has improved.

rebuilding for

Now you're into the home straight and you can see the finishing post ahead. Over the next two weeks you'll see that time and effort spent preparing and eating good food will repay itself a hundredfold in terms of your health. Unfortunately, even in the best of worlds, other things can interfere with your good intentions. What few people, even doctors, understand is that some prescribed drugs, and even medicines bought over the counter, can have damaging effects on vitamins and minerals. So if you're taking any of the following, you may need more of some foods or supplements to counteract the losses.

antacids

These interfere with vitamins A, B complex, and E, and the minerals calcium, magnesium, iron and phosphorus. Antacids containing aluminium also reduce the body's absorption of vitamin D.

antibiotics

These destroy the natural bacteria in the gut which manufacture the B vitamins. Neomycin specifically reduces the amount of B12 your body can absorb.

anti-coagulants

These include warfarin and aspirin and affect vitamin K. They are prescribed to prevent clotting so do not take extra doses of vitamin K as this will reduce their effectiveness. They can also reduce absorption of vitamin D.

anti-convulsants

These interfere with vitamins B6, D and K, and with folic acid. They're normally taken long term, for example in the treatment of epilepsy. Phenytoin (also used to treat irregular heartbeats) interferes with the absorption of calcium.

health

anti-inflammatories

These are often used for the treatment of bowel disease and may cause a loss of folic acid.

anti-ulcer drugs

These work by reducing stomach acid, but can cause poor absorption of B12.

cholesterol-lowering drugs

When used for several months continuously, these can cause poor absorption of iron, betacarotene, vitamins A, D, and K, and folic acid.

diuretics

Many of these drugs deprive the body of vitamin B complex, potassium, magnesium and zinc. Those containing slow-release potassium may have a particularly bad effect on your B12 levels.

laxatives

Regular use lowers the body's levels of calcium, iron and vitamins A, D and E. Laxative abuse can cause malnutrition and may seriously increase the risk of osteoporosis in later life.

the pill

This has an adverse effect on folic acid, and on vitamins C, E and B complex.

anti-depressants and tranquilizers

These interfere with the absorption of vitamin B2 and with the uptake of zinc and magnesium. Chronic fatigue may be caused by zinc deficiency, yet patients are often prescribed anti-depressants which lower their zinc levels even more.

fourteen-day rebuilding

For the next fortnight you start by repeating the Seven-Day Replenishing for Health programme. As I'm sure you'll remember – you have done it haven't you? – it isn't an exact eating plan but a chance to choose from a selection of health-replenishing recipes. You also need to keep going with the supplements. I know that the supplement regime may seem like a lot of pills, but it's only for another few weeks, after which you'll have rebuilt your body stores and will only need to take supplements as circumstances dictate.

After the Seven-Day Replenishing plan, you're back to an exact combination of foods for each day of the week. It's fine if you want to switch whole days around or to have the light meals and main meals at whichever time of day suits you best. But what you mustn't do is to take a light meal from one day, a main meal from another and breakfast from a third, as this will not achieve the ideal balance.

For the whole two weeks, don't exceed 14 units of alcohol a week if you're a woman, 21 for a man, and don't drink more than a total of four cups of tea and coffee in any combination you like on any one day. Canned fizzy drinks and commercial squashes are still taboo but you can drink as much herb tea, fresh unsweetened fruit juice or salt-free vegetable juice as you like. Of course you still need at least one and a half litres of water a day.

Days 1–7, follow the Seven-Day Replenishing programme.

day 8

breakfast Any porridge with a sprinkle of raisins, honey and cinnamon
Kiwi and Pineapple Juice (see recipe, page 82)

light meal Special Welsh Rarebit (see recipe, page 86)
Spinach with Yoghurt (see recipe, page 91)
A pear with a small piece of soft cheese (preferably goat's) and a bunch of red grapes

main meal Grilled Marinated Fish (see recipe, page 92) with Mixed Cabbage, Leek and Spring
Onions, (see recipe, page 92) and olive-oil mash (mashed potatoes made with olive oil – no
butter, no milk)
Yoghurt and Mango Smoothie (see recipe, page 82)

day 9

breakfast Poached Haddock with Cherry Tomatoes (see recipe, page 80)
2 thin slices unbuttered wholemeal bread
Apple, Kiwi, Pear and Celery juice (see recipe, page 83)

light meal Onion Soup (see recipe, page 102) with a chunk of wholemeal bread
Salad made of half a sliced avocado, dark green lettuce and tomato and watercress,
sprinkled with toasted sunflower seeds
A pear

main meal Chicken Jalfrezi (see recipe, page 93)
Carrot Salad (see recipe, page 103)
Any 2 pieces of fresh fruit, but not bananas

day 10

breakfast   Dutch Breakfast (see recipe, page 79)

Grape, Pear, Apple and Pineapple Juice (see recipe, page 83)

light meal   Scrambled Eggs with Smoked Mackerel (see recipe, page 93)

Watercress Salad (see recipe, page 103)

Stewed apple with live natural yoghurt

main meal   Roast Lamb with Rosemary (see recipe, page 94), Bulgur with Aubergine (see recipe, page 94) and a mixed green salad

Fresh pineapple

day 11

breakfast   Courgette and Red Leicester Omelette (see recipe, page 81)

Tomato Juice, Celery and Celery Leaf Blend (see recipe, page 82)

light meal   Pasta Noodles with Broccoli (see recipe, page 94) with a tomato and onion salad

Greek yoghurt sprinkled with chopped hazelnuts and a teaspoon of honey

main meal   Salmon in a Parcel (see recipe, page 95) with mixed green salad

Strawberries, raspberries, blueberries and a little single cream

day 12

breakfast   Sautéed Wild Mushrooms and Walnuts (see recipe, page 81) on wholemeal toast

Carrot, Apple and Celery juice (see recipe, page 83)

light meal   Devilled Sardines (see recipe, page 86) with wholemeal pitta bread and a salad of avocado and watercress sprinkled with pine nuts

Two plums

main meal   Crudités with French dressing

Spicy Chicken (see recipe, page 95) with brown rice drizzled with olive oil and some finely chopped garlic

Small piece of hard cheese and an apple

day 13

breakfast   Fresh Fruit Kebabs (see recipe, page 79)
Berry Smoothie (see recipe, page 83)

light meal   Oat and Broccoli Soup (see recipe, page 102) with a chunk of dark rye or mixed-grain bread
Mixed green salad
Piece of soft cheese, preferably goat's, with an apple

main meal   Pan-Fried Liver (see recipe, page 95) with cauliflower, broccoli and new potatoes
Thinly sliced banana sprinkled with toasted sunflower seeds, honey and a little single cream

day 14

breakfast   Porridge Muesli (see recipe, page 78)
Orange Juice and Almond Blend (see recipe, page 82)

light meal   Scrambled eggs on a bed of puréed spinach sprinkled with nutmeg
Small piece of strong Cheddar cheese and 2 sticks of celery (with leaves)

main meal   Braised Chicken (see recipe, page 96) with spring greens, dark cabbage or kale, carrots and plain boiled potatoes
A generous bowl of any berries with crème fraîche

rebuilding summary

You've now established a wonderful foundation on which to build and maintain your health for the rest of your life. Your changed eating habits are beginning to be routine for you and hopefully your whole mind-set towards food has taken on a new dimension.

When you go shopping for food, you look at things with a new perspective; when you eat in a restaurant you make different choices. However, most importantly, you have not become a food freak and you still enjoy going out with friends for a meal and having a good time.

what you've achieved

▶ You'll have a new respect for food as you realise that it's more than just fuel for your body but something which has an enormous part to play in the promotion of your good health

▶ You'll have a new appreciation and enjoyment of food, which comes from being more involved in its preparation from basic ingredients

▶ If you were one of those who worried about everything to do with eating, like calorie-counting or your fat-, salt- and sugar-intakes, that should by now be a thing of the past

▶ You'll have given yourself the basis for lifetime protection against many of the degenerative and chronic diseases of our western civilisation. You are no longer overfed yet undernourished, and you have dramatically reduced your risk of heart and circulatory disease, strokes, eye problems, high blood pressure, joint disease and with it premature disability, and death.

how you feel

▶ You should be feeling very pleased with yourself and by now you will certainly be feeling fitter and healthier

▶ You feel more self-assured as you know that you are now taking responsibility for your own health

▶ As your nutritional status improves and your immune system gets stronger, you will feel healthier and you'll get far fewer infections like coughs, colds and flu

▶ As a result of feeling better you will certainly feel more positive about life. This in itself gives even more of a boost to your natural defences, which in turn means you're even less likely to get sick

▶ One surprising consequence of completing the plan this far is that you will feel much more confident around food and with food issues. Because you'll have been doing more cooking and will have been sitting down to meals, it's more likely that you'll have been eating more meals with your family, friends, partner or spouse. Too many people have forgotten the pleasure of sharing food and conversation at the table.

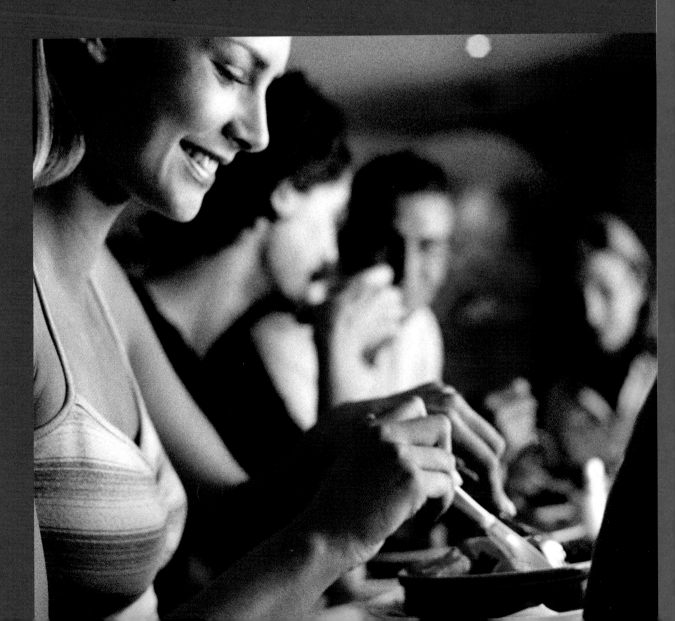

part 2

three paths to super health

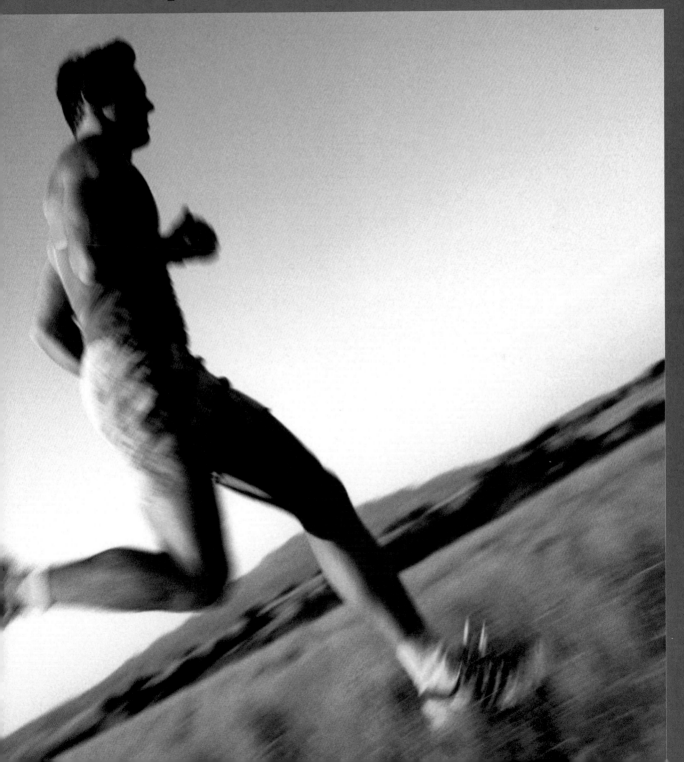

healthy eating

The first path to super health is healthy eating. 'You are what you eat' says the proverb, and of course it's true. But unfortunately, what most people don't realise is that you're also what you don't eat. In spite of the mountain of information out there about health and its relationship to nutrition, food and cooking, the messages get confused. As a result, I see in my surgery an ever-increasing number of people who are either overfed yet undernourished; or are so busy trying to follow every piece of food advice they read or hear, that they end up underfed and of course undernourished.

It's extraordinary that with the never-ending stream of cookery books that are published, the seemingly limitless number of TV shows about food, the huge amount of newspaper and magazine coverage of this topic, and the hundreds of websites devoted to food, health and nutrition, the average shopper still gets it wrong and seems unable to make sensible choices.

But how do you choose when there are so many conflicting messages? Don't eat eggs – eat eggs; eat margarine – eat butter; eat soya products – don't eat soya products; you need salt – you don't need salt; skimmed milk is healthy – full-fat milk is healthy; chocolate is good – chocolate is bad; eat meat – be a vegetarian . . . . No wonder everyone's confused and alarmed by every new report that makes the headlines. But what you must ask yourself when you read these stories is who's behind them, who stands to gain financially by putting these stories about?

It's enough to make you wonder how our great-grandparents and grandparents ever survived in the 1920s and 1930s without the army of dieticians, nutritionists (qualified and bogus), holistic health experts and lifestyle coaches that exist today. In fact, in many ways their lives were better than ours. There was less obesity, less heart disease, less cancer – and eating disorders were virtually unknown. People only ate food that was in season and mothers relied on their common sense and on the skills they'd learned from their mothers to raise healthy, well-fed families. It's just as easy to do this today. Thanks to the enormous variety of food available, it only needs a little thought to make sure you and your family get an abundance of all the essential nutrients, yet avoid the excesses that cause disease.

the three-box trick

Next time you go shopping, put three equal-sized boxes in your supermarket trolley and follow these easy rules for your one-week family food supply.

The first box should be filled to the brim with good quality carbohydrates – potatoes, rice, pasta, bread, beans, good cereals like porridge, muesli, wholegrain breakfast cereals and wholewheat flakes. The second box must overflow with fruit, vegetables and salads. You should also include dried fruits, fresh nuts and seeds. Frozen vegetables are fine if they suit your lifestyle better. They are almost as nutritious as fresh vegetables. The third box is a little more complicated. Just imagine it's divided into three compartments – two equal-sized ones that together take up 80 per cent of the space and a third occupying the last tiny 20 per cent. The first of the two equal-sized compartments contains your cheese, milk, yoghurt and eggs. The second is filled with purchases of meat, fish and poultry or with vegetarian protein such as tofu, Quorn™ or textured vegetable protein (TVP), and the final tiny space is the one where you put the cream, biscuits, sweets, chocolates, sticky buns and other treats.

Use exactly the same proportions as the basis of your daily diet when you get home. That way you'll get at least half your calories from good carbohydrates, no more than a third of them from fat, and between 10 and 12 per cent of them from protein. And by adding a couple of glasses of wine a day, your calories from alcohol will be less than 10 per cent of your daily calorie intake and won't exceed the recommended maximum number of units.

By using these proportions in your diet, you'll be eating at least five portions of fruit and vegetables a day, and so getting all the wonderful plant chemicals and antioxidants that protect you from heart disease, infections and many types of cancer. You'll also be getting more than enough protein to build and maintain strong muscles and a strong heart, and you'll get the essential fatty acids for skin, joints and hormone regulation and, according to latest research, lots of the special nutrients that reduce the risks of hay fever, asthma and other allergies. This isn't hair shirt time – you can still enjoy fresh cream on your strawberries, a piece of chocolate with your evening coffee or a delicious gooey dessert once in a while. And remember that these proportions work for everyone unless specific medical reasons dictate otherwise.

When you're shopping, buy as much fresh seasonal produce as you can and if you can find and afford organic, that's terrific, but don't become a fanatic. American paediatricians are already dealing with parents they label 'chemophobes' – people who are so obsessive about only giving their children organic food that if they can't find organic fruit and vegetables, they'd rather give them none. This is madness: the risks of depriving children of fresh produce are far greater than any risks caused by chemical residues.

Also try and use more fresh herbs in your cooking. They not only taste good but have wonderful medicinal benefits. Sage improves the digestion of fats. Mint is a powerful antacid and prevents indigestion. Basil calms you down and makes you feel good. Bay leaves are helpful for chest infections. Garlic lowers cholesterol. Coriander is good for wind and is reputedly an aphrodisiac. Dill is great for irritable bowel syndrome. Parsley is a diuretic and helps with premenstrual puffiness. And ginger is the perfect cure for early morning or travel sickness. Now just to set the record straight, here are thefacts about some of the foods you eat.

the truth about carbohydrates

Once and for all, bread, potatoes, rice, pasta and cereals are not fattening or unhealthy. It's what you do to them that makes the difference. Potatoes drizzled with olive oil, sprinkled with rosemary and roasted in the oven are wonderful. Pasta with sauce made from tomatoes, vegetables or fish is great food. Good wholemeal bread with a thin smear of butter is delicious and highly nutritious.

the truth about convenience foods

Obviously you shouldn't rely exclusively on ready-made meals, takeaways or convenience foods. Some convenience foods though, are better than others and should always be in your kitchen cupboard, for instance canned fish of all sorts, canned beans, like baked beans, kidney beans, borlotti beans and chick peas – well rinsed to remove the salt – canned tuna and tomatoes. If you always have handy some spring onions, garlic, cucumber, a pepper and your favourite salad dressing, it's easy to rustle up a healthy nourishing instant meal.

the truth about salt

Watch the labels for salt content. Salt is known to be a major factor in causing high blood pressure and strokes, so aim for 4g a day maximum – the average intake in Western countries is 12g. Once you start looking, you'll be amazed where salt crops up. Some brands of cornflakes, for example, have more salt in one bowl than the equivalent amount of seawater. So throw away the salt cellar and enjoy the wonderful flavours of the food itself, enhanced just by spices and fresh herbs.

how to gain weight & build beautiful muscles

If you're desperate to put on some weight and rebuild your health, surprisingly, the best starting point is exercise. Not aerobics, jogging or marathon running, but real old-fashioned weight training and body building. This will build bigger muscles and dramatically improve your body shape but it must go together with a dramatic increase in your good calorie consumption. What you must not do is to get these extra calories from high-sugar, high-fat foods that will make you gain weight but will dramatically increase your risks of a heart attack at the same time.

good calories

The healthiest calories come from complex carbohydrates like wholemeal bread, oats, potatoes, pasta, rice and beans. They should make up at least half of your daily food, but there is a limit to how much you can eat at one time. Get extra calories from bananas, unsalted nuts and dried fruits. Raisins, sultanas, dates and dried apricots are excellent sources of vitamins, minerals and fibre and eaten as snacks and nibbles, they add a significant number of calories in a comparatively small amount of food.

Other sources of healthy calories are seeds. Sunflower and sesame seeds are especially good, and peanut butter and tahini – a spread made from crushed sesame – provide a large number of calories, plenty of essential rebuilding nutrients and very little bulk.

grazing's ok

This is the time for you to become a grazer – aim to eat something at least every two hours, starting with a really good breakfast and finishing with a bedtime snack. Dips like guacamole, made from avocado and olive oil, or hummous, made with chickpeas and tahini, eaten with wholemeal pitta bread, make excellent between-meals snacks and like all the best foods, provide a high proportion of nutrients with their calories.

the healthy weight gain secret weapon

For all of you who suffer severe embarrassment through being underweight, here's the secret weapon in my Healthy Weight Gain Plan. It's a recipe which I've used successfully for years in my own practice. It's also excellent for anyone undergoing chemotherapy who may not feel like or be able to eat 'proper' food. Make it up first thing in the morning, drink a glass of it before breakfast, keep the rest in the fridge and make sure it's all gone by bedtime.

You'll need half a litre of whole milk, one certified salmonella-free raw egg, one banana, a dessertspoon each of molasses, honey, tahini, wheatgerm and brewer's yeast powder, and four dried apricots. Whizz all the ingredients together in a blender and enjoy.

down with obesity

The US National Center for Health Statistics reports that a third of American adults are so overweight that they exceed the maximum safe Body Mass Index. And judged by World Health Organisation standards, almost 60 per cent of men and 50 per cent of women in America would be considered at risk through being overweight or obese. In addition, the US Government now calculates that illness caused by obesity – high blood pressure, strokes, heart disease, gallstones, diabetes, cancer, arthritis – costs an annual $66 billion.

Throughout the world, the picture's similar and most alarmingly, it's the rate at which obesity has increased in children that will set the pattern for a pandemic of weight-related illnesses in coming years. In the last 25 years in the USA, the number of obese youngsters has more than trebled. Frighteningly, this effect is apparent in virtually all ethnic groups and at every socio-economic level. Even in Egypt there are nearly four times as many seriously fat children as there were 18 years ago. One worrying result of this is the growing epidemic of adult-onset or Type II diabetes – often called Non-Insulin Dependent Diabetes. This illness has always been regarded as something likely to happen in a person's late forties or fifties, but it's now showing up in children as young as eight.

Why are so many people now overweight? Although many people now consume 800 calories a day less than they did in the 1950s, we're eating 50 per cent more fat and almost everyone, including children, is far less physically active, both at work and leisure. And while the slimming industry pushes the lose-weight messages, the multinational food industry encourages an ever-increasing consumption of high-fat, high-sugar convenience and junk foods.

I'm afraid there are no magic answers to being overweight and after almost 40 years in practice, I've probably heard all the excuses – big bones, slow metabolism, glandular problems, hormone imbalance, thyroid disorders, genetic influences and the 'I hardly eat a thing so I don't know why I'm gaining weight' syndrome. Of course there are medical conditions and certain prescribed drugs which can cause weight gain and make losing weight extremely hard, but these are comparatively rare. For 90 per cent of the people

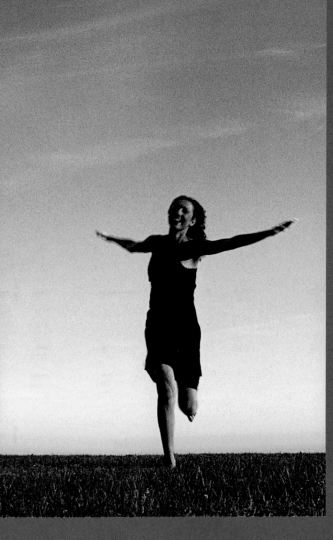

who are overweight, the answer is extremely simple. If you consume more calories than you burn, your weight goes up, and if you burn more calories than you consume, it goes down.

Here are three simple suggestions which I promise you work.

▶ If you eat two slices of bread and butter a day less and walk 15 minutes a day more, you'll lose half a kilo a week without doing anything else.

▶ If you stand up whenever you speak on the telephone, you'll lose over two kilos a year – it takes more muscle effort to stand than sit.

▶ And if you use a remote control for your TV, you'll gain a kilo a year.

There are no miracle diets, though it's true there are some that make you lose weight quickly. Unfortunately, they're either unhealthy, unsustainable or both, and the minute you stop dieting you put back on all the weight you've lost, plus a kilo or two. And each time you do that, your fat deposits move further up your body, so you gradually change from a healthy pear shape to an unhealthy apple shape – the more fat you carry around your middle, the greater the risk of heart disease.

Forget the cabbage-soup diet – it's anti-social. Forget high-protein diets – they can seriously damage your kidneys. And forget eating for your blood group, eating nothing but fruit before lunch and any other cranky diet idea that flies in the face of normal balanced eating. All you have to do to keep your weight under control is to eat good healthy food on a regular basis.

And just remember, it's what you eat most of the time that counts – what you eat occasionally doesn't matter a damn.

the ten-day weight loss plan

This ten-day eating plan is not only balanced and healthy, providing you with an excellent spread of essential nutrients, but will also help you achieve a sensible and sustainable weight loss. You can repeat the plan as many times as you like and if you're overweight, you'll lose a half to one kilo a week. You may be surprised at how much food you'll be eating every day, but don't skip any of the meals – each one is there for a purpose. It's fine to switch the days around or to switch meals on each day but this plan works best if you don't mix and match meals from different days.

There's no calorie counting, no weighing of portions. All I ask is that you use your common sense and don't go overboard when it comes to butter and oils. And you mustn't miss out on the starchy foods like pasta, rice, potatoes and bread, as these provide vital fibre, vitamins and minerals, as well as the calories needed to stimulate your metabolism and provide you with energy. This is one weight-loss plan that won't leave you feeling tired, hungry, depressed and irritable.

every day
Start every day with a large glass of hot water with the juice of half a lime – no sugar. Always eat the breakfast, and it's a good idea to take a one-a-day multivitamin and mineral supplement. Some people find it easier to eat less at a time, but more frequently. That's no problem; save some of the foods from each meal and use them as mid-morning, afternoon and late night snacks. That way you eat all the day's meals and you won't snack on forbidden 'extras'.

Drink at least one and a half litres of fluid a day, a litre of which should be water. Two cups of real coffee and two cups of tea with milk but no sugar are OK, but for other hot drinks, stick to herbal teas without milk. Although small amounts of alcohol are generally good for the health, I would advise against drinking any during this first ten days. If you decide to repeat the plan, then a couple of glasses of wine, 500ml of beer, or two pub measures of spirits twice a week are fine.

day 1

breakfast 1 whole pink grapefruit and 2 slices wholemeal toast with a very thin scraping of butter and honey

light meal Avocado, Tomato and Mushroom Salad (see recipe, page 104)

main meal Borscht (see recipe, page 100)
Grilled Chicken Breast on Iceberg lettuce (see recipe, page 85) with sweetcorn, broad beans and boiled potatoes
Fresh fruit

day 2

breakfast Poached Eggs and Tomatoes (see recipe, page 79) and 1 slice wholemeal toast with a thin scraping of butter

light meal Vegetable Soup (see recipe, page 99) and 1 wholemeal roll – no butter

main meal Grilled Marinated Fish (see recipe, page 92) with spinach and rice
A selection of ready-to-eat dried fruits

day 3

breakfast A large glass of orange juice
Porridge Muesli (see recipe, page 78)

light meal Pasta Noodles with Broccoli (see recipe, page 94)
Celery Salad (see recipe, page 104)

main meal Mixed Vegetable Stir-Fry with Rice (see recipe, page 84)
1 sliced banana sprinkled with sesame seeds and live natural yoghurt

day 4

breakfast Dutch Breakfast (see recipe, page 79)

light meal   Lettuce Soup (see recipe, page 99), 1 wholemeal roll, no butter
Selection of any fresh fruit but not bananas

main meal   Roast Lamb with Rosemary (see recipe, page ___)
Mixed Cabbage, Leek and Spring Onions (see recipe, page ___)
Fresh fruit salad of mango, kiwi and pineapple

day 5

breakfast   1 large bowl of any porridge made with half-water, half-milk, and sprinkled with raisins,
honey and cinnamon; 1 slice wholemeal toast with a thin scraping of butter
A large glass of orange juice

light meal   Grapefruit, Peach and Fromage Frais Salad (see recipe, page 105) and 2 rye crispbreads
with a thin scraping of butter

main meal   Couscous with Vegetables (see recipe, page 91)
Fresh Fruit Kebabs (see recipe, page ___)

day 6

breakfast   Yoghurt and Prune Smoothie (see recipe, page 83), 1 thick slice wholemeal toast with a
thin scraping of butter, 1 ripe banana

light meal   Tomato and Mushroom Omelette (see recipe, page 81) with a green salad

main meal   Organic Beef Stew with Vegetables (see recipe, page 91)
Natural live yoghurt with a teaspoon of honey and a generous sprinkling of toasted pine nuts

day 7

breakfast   Kiwi and Pineapple Juice (see recipe, page 82)
Natural live yoghurt with a sliced banana, fresh blueberries and honey

light meal   Tuna and Cottage-Cheese Stuffed Tomatoes (see recipe, page 88) with new potatoes

main meal Bulgur with Aubergine (see recipe, page 94)

Cucumber and Strawberry Salad (see recipe, page 103)

An apple, a pear and a matchbox-sized piece of your favourite cheese

day 8

breakfast Tomato Juice, Celery and Celery Leaf Blend (see recipe, page 82)

A bowl of any unsweetened, good quality muesli

light meal Watercress Salad (see recipe, page 103), 4 canned sardines in olive oil

2 slices wholemeal toast with a thin scraping of butter

main meal Spicy Chicken (see recipe, page 95) with tsatsiki (see recipe, page 104), rice and French beans

An orange and a bunch of grapes

day 9

breakfast Berry Smoothie (see recipe, page 83)

2 slices wholemeal toast with thinly sliced cheese and tomato – no butter

light meal Pasta with Lettuce Pesto (see recipe, page 85)

A small bunch of grapes and a kiwi fruit

main meal Pan-Fried Liver (see recipe, page 95) with mashed potato made with olive oil instead of butter, shredded cooked cabbage and Carrot Salad (see recipe, page 103)

An apple, a pear and a few grapes

day 10

breakfast Orange Juice and Almond Blend (see recipe, page 82), a banana, an apple and some grapes

light meal Falafel (see recipe, page 90) with Tomato, Red Onion and Beetroot Salad (see recipe, page 105) , a mango

main meal Oat and Broccoli Soup (see recipe, page 102)

Salmon in a Parcel (see recipe, page 95) with new potatoes and Watercress Salad (see recipe page 103)

A mixture of dried fruits and unsalted nuts

added extras for permanent protection

As you'll already have discovered, good food and regular detoxing can help promote good health and restore vitality. Sadly, our bodies have much to contend with – toxic chemical residues in food; environmental pollutants at home, at work and even in the air we breathe; extremes of stress and the ever-present threat of injury and illness.

Help insure yourself against sickness by regularly using some simple natural supplements. These added extras will give you permanent health protection.

saw palmetto

The North American Indians were the first to discover the benefits of this small palm tree. Chewing its berries not only gave their men Gladiator-style muscles, it also did wonders for their love lives. Now, a thousand years on, it is the most effective natural remedy for reducing an enlarged prostate – the uncomfortable condition caused by a swelling of the gland near the base of the penis that mainly affects men aged over 50.

green tea

Three to five cups of Japanese or Chinese green tea a day could protect you from many forms of cancer, particularly cancer of the throat. Scientists first noticed the benefits in Japan, where they drink loads of the stuff. Now, America's leading cancer organization has provided evidence that chemicals called catechins in the tea prevent the growth of tumours.

hypericum

Feeling down in the dumps isn't a twenty-first century phenomenon. Hypericum, also known as St. John's Wort, is a pretty garden plant. It has been called 'the sunshine herb' and has been used to treat psychological problems since the Middle Ages. The most recent research shows that it can treat mild to moderate depression in 70 per cent of sufferers without any side effects or risk of addiction. I've seen patients improve dramatically in two to four weeks.

added extras for permanent protection

devil's claw

Despite its unlikely nickname – its real name is the more wordy Harpagophytum procumbens – this African desert plant brings enormous relief to people suffering from arthritis and rheumatism.

It's known as Devil's Claw because of the vicious hooks on its fruits, which stick to the feet of animals or humans. I know because I trod on a few when I was out digging for it with the bushmen in the Namibian desert. They've been using it as an anti-inflammatory medicine for centuries.

selenium + vitamins A, C and E

This is a vital combination of powerful antioxidants and should always be taken during periods of increased stress, before and after surgery, after any major trauma or serious illness, and before and during prolonged periods of physical exertion. This combination provides permanent protection against damage to individual body cells and can specifically help to prevent heart disease as well as breast and prostate cancers.

glucosamine sulphate

Olympic swimmer David Wilkie was the first person to tell me about glucosamine, which he'd been given in America to relieve joint pain and keep him active. When we're young we naturally produce enough glucosamine to repair cartilage damage. The trouble starts when, as in David's case, we put extra strain on our joints, or when we get older. Glucosamine helps relieve joint pain and repair cartilage.

tea tree oil

Although the Aborigines have used tea tree oil for centuries as a treatment for cuts and wounds, it wasn't studied scientifically until the 1920s and it took another 70 years for its antiseptic and antibiotic properties to be accepted.

Use it for spots, infected nails, cold sores, dandruff, coughs, sinus problems, sore throats and other infections. Studies just published by Middlesex University in London show that tea tree oil is effective even against life-threatening antibiotic-resistant bacteria.

staying active

Staying active is the second path to super health. The best diet in the world won't help you stay healthy if you can't get up the stairs, walk to the shops or cut the grass. So if you want permanent good health, you have to exercise and keep active. This doesn't mean putting on a leotard, buying expensive trainers and sweating in a gym, nor does physical activity have to be confined to the young and beautiful. Whether you're 8 or 80, getting your body moving through regular exercise results in dramatic improvements in the way your body functions.

It builds muscle strength, which improves posture, prevents backache and reduces the pain of arthritis. It specifically improves the health and efficiency of lungs, circulation and the heart. And as your heart grows stronger it's able to pump more blood with fewer beats and less effort, which reduces the strain on the heart itself and prolongs its healthy active life.

Regular exercise also boosts your natural immunity and increases the body's resistance to disease and infection. It also makes you feel good emotionally as physical activity releases mood-boosting hormones in the brain. The most important thing is to choose an activity you enjoy and one that's appropriate to your age, ability and general health. It doesn't matter if it's walking the dog, playing bowls, windsurfing or riding a bike – half an hour, three times a week will improve your health permanently.

And remember, most fashionable exercise regimes are fine if you're fit, but are definitely not a good place to start if you're not. And if you're thinking of a personal trainer, check that they're properly qualified and know what they're doing. Aerobics, step and punchball classes, and dodgy instructors keep osteopaths like me in work.

are you fit to exercise?

Before starting any exercise programme you must assess your own fitness. If you are overweight and over 40 and you've hardly moved a muscle since you left school, seek professional advice before you start. And the same is true if you've ever been told that you have high blood pressure or heart disease. To help you decide how you stand, answer the following questions **truthfully**, then add up the number of yeses.

1   Are you over 40?

2   Is it more than 5 years since you took regular exercise?

3   Do you regularly get home and fall asleep in front of the TV?

4   Do you have any joint disease or deformity?

5   Are you more than 7kg overweight?

6   Do you ever get dizzy or faint?

7   Do you smoke?

8   Do you feel ill if you have had to run for the train?

9   Do you get out of breath easily?

10 Do you have a problem sleeping?

11 Have you ever had a serious back problem?

12 Do you drink more than 1.5 litres of beer, 3 glasses of wine or 3 spirits daily?

0-3 yeses   Good, but start exercising today

3-6 yeses   Just in time; start gently and persevere

6-12 yeses You may not make it to the gym! Get some advice before you start.

getting mobile

Fitness is a combination of strength, mobility and stamina and ideally you need all three. There's no point being strong if you can't bend down to tie your shoelace, or extremely mobile if you can't keep up with your children on a five-kilometre walk.

Staying mobile also helps you to maintain your youth and vitality. I have many patients in their eighties and nineties who I could easily take for being twenty or thirty years younger when I see them walk effortlessly into the consulting room, get themselves easily onto the treatment table or bend smoothly to pick something up from the floor.

And if you suffer from any arthritic problems, maintaining and improving your mobility is even more vital. The stiffer the affected joints become, the more painful they get and the less you can use them, which leads you into a downward spiral. There are now many studies that prove conclusively that arthritis is not a reason for inactivity. The more you exercise the joints, the more you improve your mobility, strengthen the supportive muscles and reduce the pain.

my top three exercises for mobility

▶ A good starting point for improving mobility is yoga. If you haven't exercised for a while, yoga's a safe way to start gently stretching and mobilising your joints, muscles and ligaments without the risk of injury. Yoga also provides the added bonus of improved breath control and mental as well as physical relaxation. The concentration required helps eliminate stress and anxiety, so reducing the levels of adrenaline circulating in the bloodstream. This helps to lower blood pressure and reduce the strain on the heart and blood vessels.

▶ Swimming is another excellent activity and is ideal if you spend most of your working life at a desk or in front of a computer, where poor posture maintained for long periods at a time results in a shortening of muscles, tendons and ligaments and a gradual loss of joint mobility. When you're swimming, 70 per cent of your bodyweight is supported by the water so you'll find that stiff hips and knees, rigid backs and immobile neck and shoulder joints all move far more easily when they are free from the strains of weightbearing. An added bonus is that swimming can substantially improve your breathing, so it's a particularly valuable form of exercise for asthmatics.

▶ You can combine straightforward swimming with aquarobics – specially designed exercises to do in the pool. Initially it's best to learn these in a class. Once you've mastered them, you can combine them with your regular swimming sessions.

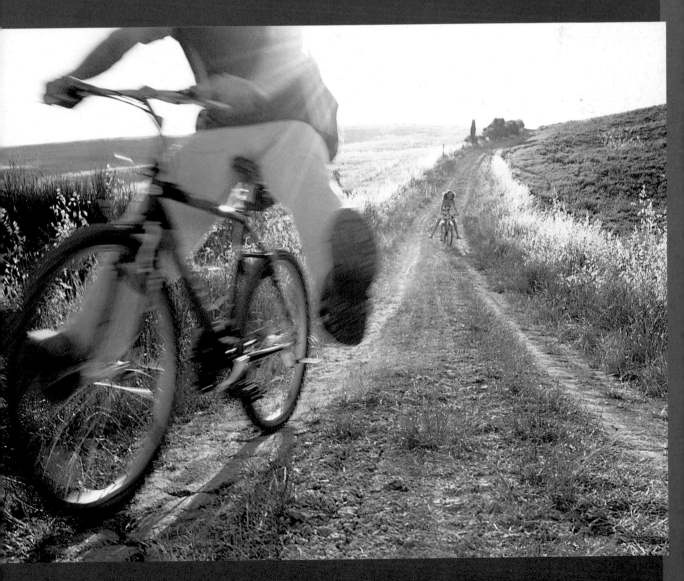

building and maintaining stamina

Once you've got mobile, building and maintaining stamina is the next step. This can only be achieved by increasing the working efficiency of your heart, circulation and lungs and by developing greater muscle strength. You do this by gradually increasing the workload of your exercise regime and extending the length of time you keep up the activity.

Always precede your exercises with a sequence of warm-ups, and end with a cool-down sequence. The warm-ups will gently stretch the muscles, speed up the circulation and increase your pulse rate. They also start the release of the body's feel-good hormones that put you in the right frame of mind for the exercise to follow. Your warm-up has got to last a minimum of five minutes and it's just as important if you're a regular athlete as it is if you're starting from scratch.

The endurance stage of your programme should last for 20–30 minutes, during which you push your heart rate up to the appropriate level (see table opposite) and keep it there. You shouldn't end up gasping for breath but as your stamina increases, you'll need to increase the length of exercise or its intensity. In the early stages, it's better to exercise less vigorously but for slightly longer periods.

The cooling-down phase is vital as it allows your heart rate and breathing to return to normal gradually, while the combination of stretching and alternate walking and jogging lets your muscles cool down slowly. You need at least six minutes in this phase.

Whatever you do, remember that your exercise regime should be fun and you mustn't allow it to become an obsession. You may find you prefer to stick to one activity, like tennis, though you'll get a better balance of strength and mobility if you do a range of different sports. A session in the gym, a session of your favourite sport and a swim is a great weekly combination. With a bit of experimentation you'll soon find what fits best with your personal preferences, work and lifestyle.

a word of warning

Great though it is to increase your activity, do not exercise if

▶ you have a heavy cold or a raised temperature

▶ you have or develop pain in the chest

▶ you have persistent joint or muscle pains for which you haven't had professional advice

▶ the weather is extremely hot or extremely cold

top tips for safe activity

Check your heart rate. Most adult men and women have a resting heart rate of 60–80 beats per minute. Find yours by pressing your wrist on the thumb side, counting the beats for 15 seconds, then multiplying by four to find the rate per minute. When you exercise, you should aim to push your heart rate up to the level recommended below.

age	beats per min
20	138–158
25	137–156
30	135–154
35	134–153
40	132–151
45	131–150
50	129–147
55	127–146
60	126–144
65	125–142
70	123–141
75	122–139
80	120–138
85	119–136

▶ When warming up and cooling down, make sure you do the stretching exercises slowly and gradually. Any short jerky movements will make your muscles contract and be more liable to damage.

▶ Don't worry if you feel a bit stiff to begin with. Your body simply isn't accustomed to exercise. These aches and pains will stop as you get fitter.

▶ Keeping well hydrated is extremely important, but stick to plain water and avoid fizzy drinks as these can make you bloated and uncomfortable. Unless you're working extremely hard, you have no need whatsoever of sports drinks or energy boosters. A banana or some dried fruits an hour before you exercise, plenty of water during your activity and more water or diluted orange juice afterwards is adequate.

▶ Remember that you're trying to train not strain, so build up your exercise gradually. One of the major risks is being too competitive and though there are people for whom winning is important, when you're building up your activity levels is not the time. Trying to keep up with a friend who's been doing aerobics classes for years, or challenging the new office junior to a game of squash when you haven't played for 20 years are both recipes for disaster.

▶ Take a shower or bath to cool down and relax your tired muscles after exercise. Take your time, don't rush and enjoy it. This is a reward for you and your muscles.

▶ I've learned from experience with my patients that it's far more effective to do your fitness routine with a partner. It's a lot more fun and if you know someone is waiting for you at the gym, the park or the swimming pool, you're more likely to keep going.

mental attitude

The third path to a healthy life is having a positive mental attitude. You can't separate the mind from the body and I've seen the effects of this relationship many times, both in my professional and my private life. Way back in the late 1950s, when I was a student, I worked as a lowly orderly in one of the world's pioneering spinal injuries centres at Stoke Mandeville Hospital near Aylesbury in Buckinghamshire.

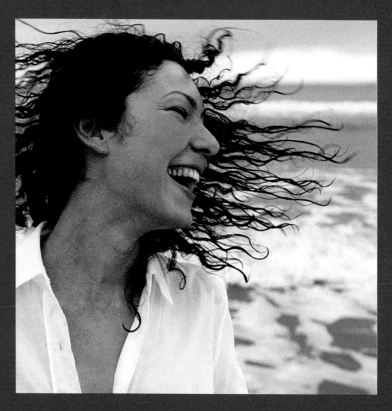

I soon learned the power of positive thought when I was looking after two young men, both paralysed from the chest down and both with identical degrees of disability. One was a soldier who'd been shot in the back, the other an affluent lawyer who'd fallen off his horse. The soldier's family was poor and lived far away, so he was on his own. The lawyer's family was rich, rented a house to be near the hospital, paid for a private room and smothered the lawyer with love and support. The soldier was desperate to be independent and was soon able to get himself off the bed, into a wheelchair and take part in the rough and tumble of wheelchair basketball. The lawyer simply turned his face to the wall and died. As it turned out, the only real difference between them was their attitude to their problem.

happiness fights disease

There's long been a suspicion that positive, happy people with a sense of inner peace are healthier than negative ones. A South African doctor once wrote a book called Happy People Don't Get Cancer – a sweeping and not wholly accurate generalisation. But it is certain that happy, positive people tend to have a stronger natural resistance to all sorts of disease. And as my story of the paralysed men shows, this happiness has little to do with material wealth.

Research at the University of Cleveland, Ohio, has now established that the mental attitude of cancer patients can make a profound difference to the outcome of their illness. In their research, patients with a positive mental attitude who saw themselves as survivors rather than victims and who played an active part in their own healing process, fared the best.

Once again, it's thanks to the complex relationship between the mental and the physical. All the evidence now shows that positive people tend to have higher levels of the special white blood cells that attack bacteria and viruses. These white blood cells are the body's first line of immune defence.

So if you're able to enjoy inner peace and happiness, whether it's through your own strength, through strong religious beliefs or simply part of your personality, you are indeed fortunate. Cultivate it, build on it and use it, because happiness is the one thing you can give away to other people without depleting your own. In fact, it's just the opposite. Sharing your happiness increases your own supply and helps promote your health to even higher levels.

think positive

Do you see your glass as half full or half empty? Yes, I know it's an old chestnut but, in the words of the comedian, the old ones are the best ones. The glass question in fact has a serious underlying message. For those who are naturally positive about life, their glass is always half full, not half empty and, as I've already said, positive equates with healthy.

People who see their glass as half empty are often those who find it impossible to take responsibility for their own actions. They believe the grass is always greener on the other side of the fence and think it's always someone else's fault they didn't get that promotion. They're convinced that the world is against them, and they end up being eaten up by negative thoughts, petty jealousies and miseries. They're no fun to be with, they're always complaining and blaming and, not surprisingly, they're nearly always ill.

combat negativity

Many sayings that have been around for years – 'smile in the face of adversity', 'look on the bright side', 'keep your chin up' – are actually exhortations to be positive. They have stood the test of time because they actually work.

One of the pioneers in the use of self-help to combat negativity was the French psychotherapist, Emile Coué. In the early 1900s he started a free clinic where he treated patients on the basis that learning to use the imagination can bring about self-healing. He encouraged his patients to repeat the now famous mantra, 'Every day and in every way I am becoming better and better', believing that if this was repeated often enough at times when the mind was most receptive, it would plant positive thoughts deep in the subconscious and these would push out the negative beliefs that were causing the unhappiness and disease.

six simple positivity-boosting exercises

Certain physical exercises can help boost your positivity and so enhance your health. Try some of these.

1 Clasp the fingers of both hands behind your head. Lift your chin and push hard against your hands for 10 seconds. Repeat 5 times.

2 Place your palms against your forehead. Try to push your chin down by pressing your head against your hands. Hold for 10 seconds. Repeat 5 times.

3 Put your left hand against the left side of head and try to push your left ear towards your left shoulder. At the same time, push your hand against the side of your head. Hold for 10 seconds. Repeat 5 times. Repeat on the right side.

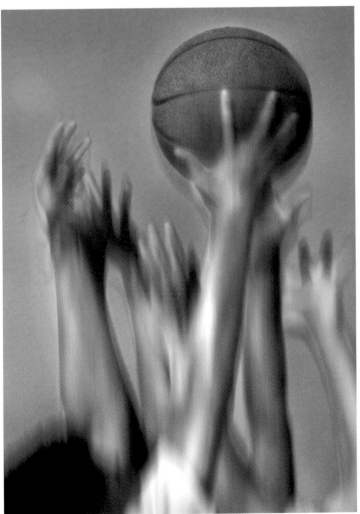

4 Standing or sitting, raise your shoulders as high as you can, with your arms hanging by your sides. Hold for 5 seconds, then let the shoulders drop with their own weight. Repeat 5 times.

5 Standing or sitting, push both shoulders back as far as you can, sticking out your chest and forcing the shoulder blades together. Hold for 5 seconds and relax. Repeat 3 times

6 Standing or sitting, push both shoulders as far forward as you can, narrowing the chest and forcing your shoulder blades as far apart as they will go, with your arms hanging down. Hold for 5 seconds and relax. Repeat 3 times.

a good night's sleep

Are you surprised to know that a bottle of milk, a spoonful of honey, a loaf of bread and a lettuce are all you need to help you to a better night's sleep? A glass of warm milk with honey is a time-honoured aid to sleep, but have it at bedtime with a lettuce sandwich and you'll be off to the land of nod before you can count ten sheep.

None of us can escape the occasional bad night. Indigestion, toothache, backache, anxiety, being too hot or too cold, a snoring partner . . . these are just some of the things that can conspire to rob us of our beauty sleep.

But real insomnia is a state of habitual sleeplessness repeated night after night, often for months or even years on end. On top of that, worrying about the insomnia, often to the point of obsession, does more damage than the lack of sleep itself. But there's no need to limp through the rest of your life on the crutch of sleeping pills, tranquillisers or alcohol.

my top tips for a good night's rest

▶ **What you eat before bedtime is key.** Going to bed too full or too hungry both interfere with sleep. Avoid eating too late, especially foods high in animal protein. This type of food is high in the amino acid tyrosine, which triggers the production of activity hormones. Starchy food, on the other hand, encourages the body to produce serotonin, the brain chemical that has a calming effect on the brain and nervous system. This is why the lettuce sandwich really does have a basis in science.

Z Z Z

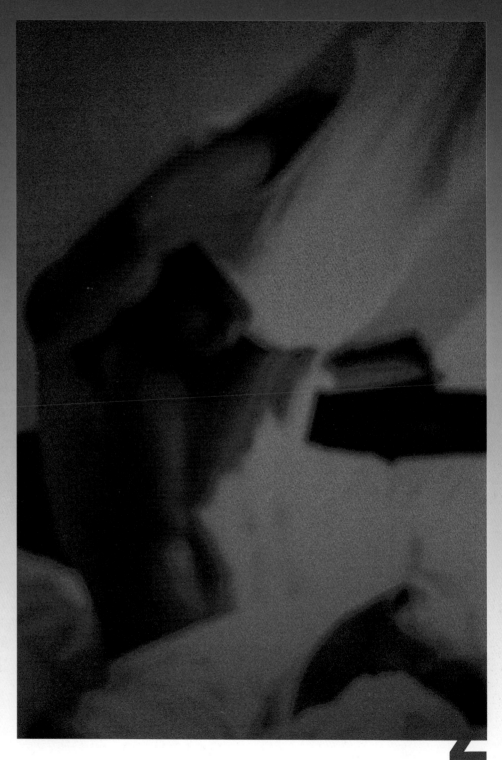

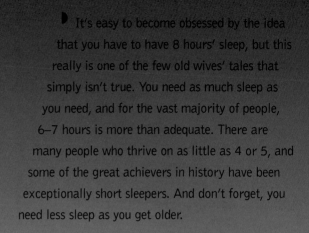

It's easy to become obsessed by the idea that you have to have 8 hours' sleep, but this really is one of the few old wives' tales that simply isn't true. You need as much sleep as you need, and for the vast majority of people, 6–7 hours is more than adequate. There are many people who thrive on as little as 4 or 5, and some of the great achievers in history have been exceptionally short sleepers. And don't forget, you need less sleep as you get older.

Finally, if you really can't sleep, don't just lie there worrying. Get up and do some of the boring chores you need to catch up on – the ironing, writing a shopping list, clearing out the cutlery drawer, paying those unpaid bills. Don't turn on the television and watch the midnight thriller, and don't start reading the latest bestseller or you'll be there till dawn. Do something dull and you'll soon find that bed beckons.

natural aids to a good night's sleep

These herbal remedies are non-addictive, don't disturb your natural sleep patterns and won't leave you feeling like you've got a hangover next morning. Because they're gentler than conventional drugs they don't work instantly and you may need to persevere for a few nights before you get maximum benefit.

Extract of passiflora promotes natural sleep. It's perfect if you get to sleep without any problems but keep waking during the night.

A standardized extract of valerian calms and soothes away the stresses of a hectic life. It's the answer for people who find it hard getting off to sleep.

Lime-blossom tea with added honey.

leisure = pleasure = health

Believe it or not, in England there's a scientific body called ARISE. Some of their prestigious meetings include lavish dinners where many different wines are served with each course, and the diners eat foie gras, goose, chocolate pudding, cheese and petits fours. Then they are encouraged to enjoy a large Havana cigar with their port and the meal finishes with strong black coffee.

Appalling? No, because ARISE is an acronym for Associates for Research Into the Science of Enjoyment. Like me, its members are increasingly concerned that the 'food and health police' are creating a world where enjoyment and pleasure stand for sin and guilt. We've seen earlier how important a positive attitude is in the creation and preservation of good health, and I can't repeat too often that as far as nutrition is concerned, it's what you do most of the time that's important, while what you do occasionally is of little consequence. Little consequence except, that is, when what you do occasionally gives you pleasure. And for the benefit of your health, pleasure should be the object of your leisure time.

The reasons for this are not just psychological. When you're stressed — as so many of us are these days — the constant over-production of adrenaline increases your heart rate speeds your respiration and increases your blood pressure. Enjoyable activities counteract all these adverse physiological effects.

In addition, quality leisure time spent with your family and friends is essential for mind, body and spirit. It's vital to the building and maintenance of good relationships. When your children leave home, it's too late to regret the sports days you missed, the school plays you never went to and the holidays you never had together. Unfortunately, the pressures of today's life are such that people find it increasingly difficult to set aside time for leisure.

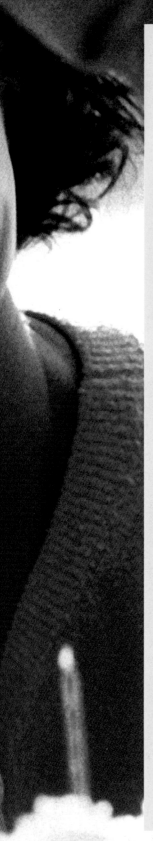

the enemies of leisure

The two great enemies of healthy leisure time are the television and the computer. Falling asleep in front of the evening movie the minute you've finished your meal, or spending three hours after work on the internet will not rebuild your health. It's not that long ago that the worst punishment for a child was being sent to its room but today, getting them out of their bedroom and away from the computer and games console is a major problem.

If you really want to give your health a boost, there are far better ways to spend your leisure time.

▶ Holidays. You may find that taking a long holiday can create almost more stress than remaining at work. A long holiday requires complex planning, and then you may worry constantly while you're away about the work still to be done and that you'll return to a bigger workload than ever. If this happens, it's often more beneficial to take 3- or 4-day breaks. But don't take your mobile phone and laptop with you, or leave a dozen contact numbers with the office. As you'd soon discover if you were made redundant, no-one is indispensable and if the business can't function without you for a while, then you and others are not doing the job properly.

▶ Learn a new skill. It may sound trite to say join the local dramatic society, go to painting classes, or learn a foreign language. But these are great ways of meeting new non-work-related people and of participating in activities which require a different set of skills. All this will help you take your mind off the trials and tribulations of your working life.

▶ Involve the family. If you have a family then some of your leisure activities must involve them too. It doesn't matter whether it's following a football team, going camping, doing jigsaw puzzles or playing Scrabble together. Activities like these not only represent a huge investment in your physical health, but are an important supportive prop for the emotional health and wellbeing of your family unit.

▶ Make sure you're really having fun. Many people, even when they do make time in their busy schedules for leisure activities, are so afraid that they might be seen to be enjoying themselves that they fill this time with punishing exercise regimes, obsessional competitive games or 'team-building' activities. This is not leisure for pleasure and does nothing to improve your health. In fact the reverse is true.

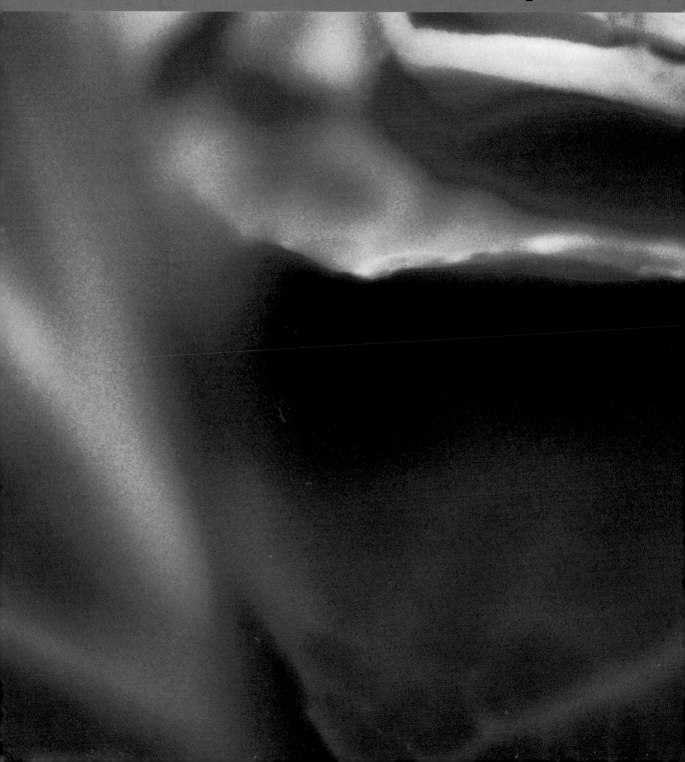

part 3

eat your way to super health

all recipes serve 4, except drinks recipes which serve 2

bread and breakfast

my easy bread

stoneground organic wholemeal bread flour	700g
easy-blend dried yeast	1 x 7g sachet
extra-virgin olive oil	2 tsp, plus extra for oiling
molasses, dark muscovado sugar or honey	1 tsp
salt	½ tsp
warm water	600ml
sunflower seeds (optional)	2 tbsp

Good bread is a vital part of any healthy diet, but most commercial bread contains added chemicals that you don't want, as well as far too much salt, which causes fluid retention and reduces the body's natural cleansing and detoxing abilities. The answer is to make your own.

Lightly oil a 1kg loaf tin and keep it warm. Mix the flour and yeast together in a large bowl. Dissolve the olive oil, molasses, sugar or honey and salt in the water. Make a well in the centre of the flour and pour in the warm water mixture and sunflower seeds, if using.

Mix all the ingredients together with a wooden spoon, then knead for about 4 minutes, until the dough forms a ball. Put it into the warm tin, cover with a damp tea towel and leave to rise in a warm place for about 40 minutes or until it has risen almost to the top of the tin. Meanwhile, preheat the oven to 200°C/400°F/Gas 6.

Transfer the tin to the preheated oven and bake for about 40 minutes, until it sounds hollow when you tap the bottom of the tin. When it's ready, remove from the oven and when it's cool enough to handle, transfer to a wire rack to cool completely.

porridge muesli

porridge oats	8 heaped tbsp
raisins	4 heaped tsp
apples	2 large
lemon	juice of ½
single cream	4 tbsp

Put the oats into a bowl. Add the raisins and about 6 tbsp of cold water. Cover with clingfilm and leave overnight. Before serving in the morning, grate the apple into the bowl, add the lemon juice and stir in the cream.

poached eggs and tomatoes

cider or white wine vinegar	1 tsp
tomatoes	4
eggs	4
wholemeal bread	4 slices
butter	for spreading

Fill a large, deep-sided frying pan with water. Add the vinegar – it helps stop the egg whites from 'fraying'. Add the whole tomatoes to the pan, bring to the boil and reduce to a simmer. Roll the eggs, in their shells, in the water for about 15 seconds – again to keep the whites intact. Break the eggs into the water and continue simmering for about 4 minutes. Meanwhile, toast the bread and butter it. Using a slotted spoon, remove the eggs from the water and place on the toast. Remove the tomatoes with a slotted spoon, rub off their skins and serve with the eggs and toast.

fresh fruit kebabs

wooden skewers	4
pineapple	1, small, peeled and cubed
black grapes	about 100g, large, seedless
apple	1, cored and cubed
pears	2, cored and cubed
runny honey	4 tbsp
ground cloves	4 pinches

Simple, impressive and wonderfully healthy as part of your detox regime.

Soak the skewers in water for 30 minutes before using to prevent burning. Preheat the grill to high and line a grill pan with foil. Make sure the pieces of fruit are roughly the same size and thread them on to the skewers. Put the kebabs on the foil-lined grill pan, drizzle with the honey and sprinkle with the ground cloves. Cook under a very hot grill for 2 minutes, then serve.

dutch breakfast

wholemeal bread	4 slices
butter	for spreading
Gouda cheese	4 thin slices
tomatoes	4, thinly sliced

As half a Dutchman, I grew up sharing this typical breakfast with my father. It's worth getting a cheese slicer, though you can buy ready-sliced packs of good Dutch cheese. Cheese contains health-giving calcium, protein, vitamin C and fibre and this recipe is very quick to make.

Simplicity itself . . . just toast the bread and spread with the butter. Top with the cheese slices, then the tomatoes and serve.

poached haddock with cherry tomatoes

whole or semi-skimmed milk	about 425ml
butter	50g
undyed smoked haddock fillets	4, weighing about 175g each
cherry tomatoes	12
black pepper	to season
parsley, to garnish	4 large sprigs

Haddock is a wonderful source of protein and minerals, particularly iodine, which is frequently deficient in most diets. Iodine controls the thyroid gland, which is not only essential for good health, but the key to effective detoxing as it stimulates the metabolism.

Fill a large, deep-sided frying pan with the milk. Add the butter and bring to the boil. Place the fish in the pan and simmer for 5–7 minutes, depending on the thickness of the fish. Add the cherry tomatoes 1 minute before the end of the cooking time to warm through. Drain the fish and tomatoes and transfer to a serving plate. Season with generous twists of coarsely ground black pepper and garnish with the parsley.

kedgeree

rice	110g wholegrain, long-grain
cod or undyed smoked haddock	110g, freshly poached, flaked, with skin and bones removed
semi-skimmed milk	enough to poach the fish
prawns (optional)	8, large, ready-cooked and peeled
curry powder	1 tsp
parsley	1 tbsp finely chopped leaves
lemon	juice of ½
butter	25g
eggs	2

Rinse the rice and cook according to the packet instructions. Meanwhile, put the fish into a large, deep-sided frying pan, add enough milk to cover and bring slowly to the boil. As soon as it begins to boil, remove from the heat. Cover and leave for 10 minutes. Remove the fish from the pan with a slotted spoon, then skin and flake it, removing all the bones. While the rice is cooking, poach the eggs.

Drain the rice thoroughly and fluff up with a fork. While it's still warm, gently stir in the prawns, flaked fish, curry powder, most of the parsley, lemon juice and butter. Transfer the rice mixture to serving plates, arrange a poached egg on top and sprinkle with the remaining parsley. Serve immediately.

tomato and mushroom omelette

butter	75g
tomatoes	8, medium, roughly chopped
mushrooms	110g, closed-cap, wiped and roughly chopped
eggs	10
basil	4 heaped tbsp roughly torn leaves

Melt the butter in a large omelette or nonstick frying pan. Add the tomatoes and mushrooms, cover and simmer gently for 10 minutes. Remove the vegetables with a slotted spoon and reserve until required. Beat the eggs, pour a quarter of the mixture into the pan, drawing the mixture in from the sides and tilting the pan to make sure you have an even layer. As soon as the omelette begins to set, add a quarter of the tomato and mushroom mixture and swirl around to make sure it is evenly distributed. Cook for 1–2 minutes to brown underneath. Slide the omelette onto a serving plate and sprinkle with half of the basil leaves. Repeat to make the other 3 omelettes.

courgette and red leicester omelette

butter	25g
eggs	8, large
courgettes	2 medium, grated
red Leicester cheese	110g, grated
cucumber	½, peeled and finely sliced

Melt the butter in a large omelette or nonstick frying pan over a low heat. Beat 4 of the eggs and add to the pan. As soon as the omelette begins to set, sprinkle half the courgettes and cheese on top. Continue cooking over a low heat until the cheese has melted. Fold the omelette in half, cut into 2 and serve with the cucumber. Repeat to make a second omelette.

sautéed wild mushrooms and walnuts

walnut oil	3 tbsp
butter	25g
wild mushrooms	175g, wiped and cut into about 1cm slices
walnuts	50g, chopped
Little Gem lettuce	1, trimmed and chopped
soft goat's cheese	100g, cut into small cubes

For breakfast, brunch or even a light supper, this is a great recipe. Rich in mono-unsaturated fats from the walnuts and walnut oil, which help eliminate cholesterol and protect the heart and circulation. Easily digested and perfect as a post-detox returning to normal meals.

Melt the walnut oil and butter gently in a large frying pan over a low heat. Add the mushrooms and walnuts, cover the pan and simmer gently for 10 minutes. Arrange the lettuce on 2 serving plates. Using a slotted spoon, remove the mushrooms and walnuts from the pan and arrange over the lettuce. Scatter on the goat's cheese and top with the juices from the frying pan. Serve immediately.

drinks

When detoxing and fasting, keeping your fluid levels up is even more important than in day-to-day life. The drinks in this section all provide a health bonus on top of their liquid content.

For juicing, most produce only needs washing and cutting into small enough pieces to fit into the machine. There's normally no need to peel or remove the core, but obviously you must take out any stones. Thick skins, like those on mangoes and pineapples, usually need to be removed. Ideally, use organic produce wherever possible. There are no rules, just experiment with whatever you have in stock to find your favourite combos.

tomato juice, celery and celery leaf blend

plum tomatoes	6 large, ripe
celery	2 stalks, with leaves
lemon	juice of 1
Tabasco (optional)	a dash

Simply put the tomatoes, celery and lemon juice in a blender or food processor and blend until smooth. Season to taste with the Tabasco sauce.

orange juice and almond blend

oranges	4 large, juiced
ground almonds	4 tbsp

Simply mix the two ingredients together and whisk with a fork.

kiwi and pineapple juice

kiwi fruit	4, ripe, peeled
pineapple	1, medium, top removed

Just cut the fruit into pieces and juice. Some of the heavy-duty juicers will cope with fruit with a tough skin like pineapples. Check your machine's instructions.

yoghurt and mango smoothie

live natural yoghurt	300g
mango	1, large, ripe, peeled and cubed

Put the ingredients into a blender or liquidizer and whizz until smooth.

apple, kiwi, pear and celery juice

apples, preferably Cox's	3, quartered
kiwi fruit	3, ripe, peeled
pears	2
celery	2 stalks, with leaves

Put the ingredients in a blender and whizz until smooth.

grape, pear, apple and pineapple juice

grapes	110g, black, seedless
pears	3
apples, preferably Cox's	3, quartered
pineapple	½, large

Put the ingredients in a blender and whizz until smooth.

berry smoothie

mixed fresh berries	200g, hulled
live natural yoghurt	300g
lemon	zest of ½
ground cinnamon	½ level tsp
fresh mint	2 sprigs, to garnish

Put the ingredients into a blender or liquidizer and whizz until smooth.

yoghurt and prune smoothie

live natural yoghurt	400g
prunes	12, stoned

Put the ingredients into a blender or liquidizer and whizz until smooth.

carrot, apple and celery juice

carrots	3, large, topped and tailed, and peeled if not organic
apples	2, quartered
celery	2 stalks

Simply cut into pieces and juice.

parsley tea

Put 2 heaped tbsp chopped fresh parsley into a large jug. Add 500ml of boiling water, cover and leave to stand for 10 minutes. Strain, cool and keep covered in the fridge.

ginger tea

Add 2.5cm fresh grated root ginger to a mug of boiling water. Cover and leave to stand for 5 minutes. Strain, add 1 tsp of honey and sip slowly.

lunches and dinners

mixed vegetable stir-fry with rice

With such a wide variety of vegetables, this is an amazingly protective dish full of resistance-boosting nutrients.

sesame oil	2 tbsp
rapeseed oil	2 tbsp
carrots	2, in julienne strips
broccoli	12 small florets
celery	2 stalks, finely sliced
spring onions	4, cut diagonally
mangetout	75g, quartered
baby sweetcorn	75g, in 1cm chunks
fresh peas	75g
basmati rice	110g
very veggie stock (see recipe, page 97)	about 1 litre
light soy sauce	2 tsp

Heat the oils in a preheated wok or large frying pan. Add the vegetables and cook over a medium heat for 5 minutes, stirring continuously, until just **al dente**. Meanwhile, cook the rice in a saucepan of boiling water according to the packet instructions. Pour the stock into the vegetables and boil rapidly until most of the liquid is absorbed. Add the soy sauce, mix thoroughly and serve the vegetables over the rice.

home-made chicken liver pâté

This may seem an unhealthy inclusion for a health detox book, but it's a far cry from commercially made pâtés. Yes, it does contain butter, cream and brandy, but it's also full of iron, B vitamins – especially B12 – and all the cleansing properties of garlic, onions and parsley. Indulge.

unsalted butter	60g
onion	1, very finely chopped
garlic	2 cloves, very finely chopped
chicken livers	500g, fresh or frozen, washed and with membranes removed
single cream	3 tbsp
tomato purée	1 tbsp
brandy	2 tbsp
bay leaves	3
parsley	1 tbsp freshly chopped leaves

Melt half the butter in a large frying pan and sauté the onion and garlic gently for 3 minutes. Add the chicken livers and continue cooking gently for 5 minutes, stirring continuously, until soft but not browned. Transfer to a bowl and mash thoroughly with a fork. Pour in the cream, tomato purée and brandy and mix again, adding more cream if the mixture seems too thick. Spoon into a half-litre terrine or other suitable dish and refrigerate.

When the pâté is cool and set, melt the rest of the butter in a small saucepan. Place the bay leaves on the pâté, sprinkle the parsley on top, pour over the melted butter and return to the fridge until the butter is set.

pasta with lettuce pesto

A wonderfully healthy pasta, providing energy, calcium and protein, plus calming natural chemicals to help you unwind and sleep.

fusilli	400g
radicchio	1 large head, washed
pine kernels	25g
extra-virgin olive oil	4 tbsp
Parmesan cheese	4 tbsp, freshly grated
white lettuce	1 small handful, leaves roughly torn

Cook the pasta in a large saucepan of boiling water according to the packet instructions. Meanwhile, put the radicchio, pine kernels and half the oil into a food processor and whizz until smooth. Keeping the machine running, add the rest of the oil in a gentle stream. When thoroughly blended, pour into a bowl and stir in the cheese and lettuce. Stir the pesto into the pasta and serve.

grilled chicken breast on iceberg lettuce

chicken breasts	4, skinless, boneless and flattened slightly
lime	juice of 1
extra-virgin olive oil	2 tbsp
garlic	1 clove, finely chopped
tarragon	4 sprigs
Iceberg lettuce	1 medium

Preheat the grill. Put the chicken breasts into a large, shallow dish. Mix the lime juice, olive oil and garlic together in a separate bowl and pour over the chicken. Add the tarragon and stir until the chicken is well coated in the marinade. Cover with clingfilm and leave in the fridge for at least 1 hour.

Drain the chicken, reserving the marinade. Put the chicken on a grill pan and cook under the grill for 15 minutes, turning once. Meanwhile, shred the lettuce and warm the rest of the marinade gently in a small saucepan. Serve the chicken on the lettuce, drizzled with the warmed marinade.

mushrooms with radicchio and chicory

butter	50g, unsalted
mushrooms	4, large, wiped and peeled
chicory	2 heads
wholemeal bread	4 thick slices
radicchio	1 bunch

Melt the butter in a large heavy-bottomed pan until soft. Add the mushrooms, cover the pan and cook over a medium heat for 10 minutes. Remove from the heat and transfer to a foil-lined grill pan. Cook under a gentle grill until the juices begin to run. Brush the chicory leaves with the butter from the mushrooms, and put under the grill until wilted. Divide the bread between 4 serving plates, arrange the radicchio on top, the charred chicory around the edges, then add the mushrooms and serve.

devilled sardines

fresh sardines	4, cleaned
Dijon mustard	2 tbsp
cayenne pepper	1 tsp
wholemeal bread	4 slices
tomatoes	2 slices
lemon	1, quartered

I cannot emphasize too often the importance of oily fish. They're a natural anti-inflammatory and essential during pregnancy and breastfeeding for the growing baby's brain development. They are also the richest source of vitamin D – needed to turn calcium into strong bones.

Preheat the grill and line the grill rack with foil. Make diagonal cuts in the sardines and rub with the mustard. Sprinkle the cayenne pepper on both sides. Cook under the preheated grill for 5 minutes, turning once. Meanwhile, toast the bread. Serve the sardines with the toast, tomatoes and lemon quarters.

special welsh rarebit

mature Cheddar cheese	175g, grated
full-fat milk	3 tbsp
Worcestershire sauce	1 tsp
Dijon mustard	1 tsp
paprika	1 pinch
parsley	2 tsp freshly chopped leaves
wholemeal bread	4 thick slices

A slice of processed cheese grilled on a piece of bread isn't a Welsh rarebit. Try this recipe instead – it contains lots of healing nutrients, has a great flavour and only takes a few minutes.

Preheat the grill and line a grill pan with foil. Mix the cheese and milk together. Add the Worcestershire sauce, mustard, paprika and half the parsley and stir again until completely combined. Toast the bread on one side, turn it over and arrange the cheese mixture on top. Return to the grill and cook until the cheese bubbles. Serve with the extra parsley scattered on top.

ratatouille

extra-virgin olive oil	6 tbsp
onions	2, large, finely chopped
garlic	4 cloves, finely chopped
green peppers	2, large, deseeded and finely chopped
aubergine	1, large, finely cubed
chopped tomatoes	1 x 400g can

Heat the olive oil and sauté the onions and garlic gently for 5 minutes in a large saucepan. Add the peppers and aubergine and continue to sauté for a further 5 minutes. Add the tomatoes, cover the pan and simmer gently for 30 minutes.

baked stuffed trout

Trout is another wonderful oily fish. Need I say more?

extra-virgin olive oil	4 tbsp
onion	1, large, finely chopped
garlic	2 cloves, finely chopped
butter beans	1 x 200g can, rinsed and mashed
spinach	175g, thoroughly washed and roughly torn
salmon trout	4, cleaned
dry white wine	1 large glass
unsalted butter	75g
lemon	1, large, sliced

Preheat the oven to 220°C/425°F/ Gas 7. Heat the olive oil in a saucepan and sauté the onion and garlic gently for 5 minutes. Drain off any excess oil. Mix them into the mashed beans and spinach. Cut 4 pieces of foil large enough to make a parcel round each fish. Lay a fish on each piece of foil and fill each fish cavity with the bean and spinach mixture. Pour a quarter of the wine over each. Dot with the butter and top with a slice of lemon. Fold the foil over and tuck in the ends. Place the parcels on baking sheets and cook for 20 minutes.

veggie curry with rice

At first sight, you may not think of curry as part of a healthy detox plan, but you'd be wrong. Apart from the cleansing and health-promoting vegetables, the turmeric in curry paste is a valuable anti-cancer spice.

extra-virgin olive oil	6 tbsp
onion	1, large, finely sliced
garlic	2 cloves, finely chopped
chilli	1, small, red, deseeded and finely chopped
fresh root ginger	1cm, peeled and grated
green Thai curry paste	1 heaped tbsp
cauliflower	10 florets
carrots	3, in fine julienne strips
potatoes	2, new, in 1cm cubes
parsnips	1, peeled, in 1 cm cubes
turnips	1, peeled, in 1 cm cubes
very veggie stock (see recipe, page 97)	500ml
coconut milk	400ml
basmati rice	110g

Heat the oil in a large saucepan and gently soften the onion, garlic, chilli and ginger for 5 minutes. Add the curry paste and stir until completely combined. Add the cauliflower, carrots, potatoes, parsnips and turnips and stir continuously for a further 10 minutes. Pour in the stock and coconut milk and simmer for 40 minutes until all the vegetables are tender.

Meanwhile, cook the rice according to the packet instructions. Serve the rice with the vegetable curry on top.

tuna and cottage-cheese stuffed tomatoes

beef tomatoes	8, large, sliced widthways, membranes and pips removed
tuna	1 x 200g can in olive oil, drained
cottage cheese	1 x 200g tub
capers	2 tbsp, soaked in milk for 5 mins, then drained
chives	10 snipped, 4 left whole
black pepper	to taste

Put the tomatoes into a wide, shallow dish. Mix the drained tuna, cottage cheese, capers and snipped chives together in a bowl. Season to taste with black pepper. Pile the cheese mixture into the tomato hollows. Garnish with the remaining chives and serve.

stir-fried tofu with vegetables and noodles

lime	juice of 1
mango	1, peeled and finely cubed
Tabasco sauce	½ tsp
garlic	2 cloves, finely chopped
tofu	1 x 250g packet, drained and cubed
onion	1, medium, finely chopped
extra-virgin olive oil	2 tbsp
instant noodles	75g
kale	175g, finely chopped
beansprouts	275g

Most carnivores eat far too much meat. Good meat, preferably organic, in modest quantities, is great food if you like it. But too much has been linked to bowel cancer, raised cholesterol and high blood pressure. Here's your chance to use tofu, a soy product that's rich in natural plant hormones and extremely healthy.

Preheat the oven to 220°C/425°F/Gas 7. Mix the lime, mango, Tabasco sauce and half the garlic together in a bowl. Put the tofu into a shallow dish, add the marinade and stir to coat. Cover with clingfilm and refrigerate for 30 minutes. Transfer the tofu and marinade to the preheated oven and cook for 20 minutes.

Meanwhile, sauté the onion and remaining garlic in the oil in a wok or large frying pan for 5 minutes. In another pan, cook the noodles according to the packet instructions, usually 2–3 minutes. Add the kale and beansprouts to the onion mixture and stir until just wilted. Drain the noodles, add to the wok and cook for a further 2 minutes. Add the tofu with its marinade and stir gently before serving.

pasta all'aglio e olio

This dish is great for both its energy-giving and health-boosting properties. The garlic lowers cholesterol, reduces blood pressure and makes blood less likely to clot, as well as being antibacterial and antifungal.

spaghettini	400g
extra-virgin olive oil	6 tbsp
garlic	3 cloves, peeled and crushed with the flat blade of a broad knife
Parmesan cheese	4 tbsp, freshly grated
fresh basil	6 large sprigs, leaves removed and finely torn

Cook the pasta according to the packet instructions. Meanwhile, heat the olive oil in a saucepan, add the garlic and cook gently until just beginning to turn brown. Remove the garlic with a slotted spoon and discard. Pour the hot oil over the pasta and mix thoroughly. Stir in the Parmesan cheese and mix again. Finally, stir in the basil leaves and serve immediately.

grilled salmon steak

salmon steaks	4
extra-virgin olive oil	6 tbsp
black pepper	to taste
tarragon	8 sprigs; 4 whole, 4 with the leaves torn off and finely chopped
unsalted butter	75g, softened

Put the salmon steaks into a wide casserole dish. Pour over the olive oil and season to taste with freshly ground black pepper. Add the whole tarragon sprigs. Turn the salmon over carefully in the dish to marinate, cover with clingfilm and refrigerate for 1 hour. Meanwhile, mix the chopped tarragon into the softened butter and put it into the fridge to harden.

Preheat the grill to high and line the grill pan with foil. Remove the salmon from the marinade, leaving some of the oil clinging. Cook the fish under the preheated grill for 6–7 minutes, turning once. Serve with the tarragon butter on top.

baked leeks with cheese and eggs

baby leeks	16, cleaned and trimmed, but with most of the green parts if they're tender
single cream	200ml
eggs	3
Emmental cheese	100g, grated
salt and black pepper	to taste
parsley	3 tbsp finely chopped leaves

Preheat the oven to 200°C/400°F/Gas 6. Put the leeks into a saucepan of boiling water and simmer for 5 minutes. Drain carefully and place in an oblong casserole. Whisk the cream, eggs and half the cheese together. Season to taste. Pour the mixture over the leeks and sprinkle the rest of the cheese over the top. Bake in the preheated oven for 15 minutes, until the cheese is golden and beginning to bubble. Serve sprinkled with the parsley.

falafel

chickpeas	2 x 400g cans, drained and rinsed well
extra-virgin olive oil	4 tbsp
onion	1, large, finely chopped
garlic	2 cloves, finely chopped
parsley	4 tbsp finely chopped leaves
allspice	5 tsp
baking powder	½ tsp
rapeseed oil	about 200ml
Iceberg lettuce	1, shredded

This classic Middle Eastern dish is another meat-free treat, with no saturated fat or cholesterol, lots of calcium and plenty of protein.

Put the chickpeas and olive oil into a blender or food processor and whizz until smooth. Add the onion, garlic, parsley, allspice and baking powder and whizz again. Transfer the mixture to a bowl and form into small burger-type shapes, about 2cm across. Place on a flat plate and leave in the fridge for 30 minutes.

Heat the rapeseed oil in a large frying pan and fry the falafel for about 2 minutes on each side. Drain on kitchen paper. Serve on a bed of Iceberg lettuce.

pheasant casserole with red cabbage

for the pheasant casserole

pheasants	2, cleaned and with any shot removed
garlic	6 cloves, sliced
lemon	1
thyme	4 large sprigs
extra-virgin olive oil	2 tbsp
onion	1, finely sliced
carrots	2, sliced

for the red cabbage

extra-virgin olive oil	4 tbsp
onion	1, finely sliced
garlic	2 cloves, finely chopped
red cabbage	1, medium, finely sliced
cider vinegar	4 tbsp
brown sugar	1 tbsp

People often consider game as a 'rich meat'. Nothing could be further from the truth as pheasant, like all game, is extremely low in fat, but rich in iron and B vitamins. With the red cabbage, you get all the traditional protection and health promotion of this king of vegetables.

Preheat the oven to 180°C/350°F/Gas 4. Make several incisions into the flesh of the pheasants and insert the sliced garlic cloves. Rub the skins with the lemon and put the thyme inside the cavities. Heat the oil in a heavy-based casserole and sauté the onion and carrots for 5 minutes, then remove from the casserole and reserve. Add the pheasants and brown on all sides. Add the reserved onions and carrots. Cover and cook in the preheated oven for 45 minutes until the juices run clear when a skewer is inserted into the thickest part of the thigh.

Meanwhile, cook the cabbage. Heat the oil in a saucepan and sauté the onion and garlic gently. Stir in the cabbage and add the vinegar and sugar. Transfer to a casserole dish, cover and cook with the pheasants for the last 30 minutes of cooking time.

Serve the pheasants with the red cabbage and with the onion and carrots, which will have made a wonderfully flavoured purée.

couscous with vegetables

olive oil	4 tbsp
onion	1, finely sliced
leek	1, trimmed and finely sliced
carrots	2, diced
celery	2 stalks, finely sliced
mushrooms	110g, finely sliced
dried fruit	110g, mixed sultanas, raisins and apricots
couscous	400g

Snip the apricots to the size of the raisins. Heat the oil in a saucepan and sauté the onions gently until soft. Add the other vegetables and the dried fruit, cover and cook gently until tender – about 15 minutes. Add water if it seems to be drying out. Meanwhile, bring 500ml of water to the boil in a large saucepan. Add the couscous, reduce the heat and cook for 1 minute, stirring continuously. Remove from the heat, cover and leave for 5 minutes until all the water is absorbed. Stir in the vegetables and dried fruit and serve.

organic beef stew with vegetables

rapeseed oil	4 tbsp
onion	1, finely sliced
garlic	2 cloves, peeled and finely chopped
organic plain flour	3 heaped tbsp
herbes de Provence	1 level tbsp
lean organic braising steak	450g, cubed
very veggie stock (see recipe, page 97)	1 litre
carrots	2, finely sliced
turnip	1, cubed
parsnip	1, in julienne strips
celery	2 stalks, sliced
bay leaves	2
rice or mashed potato	to serve

If you're going to eat beef occasionally, splash out and go organic. It tastes better, contains less saturated fat and much more of the health-promoting fat CLA (conjugated linoleic acid), which is essential for the breakdown of other fats.

Heat the oil gently in a pan and sauté the onion and garlic for 5 minutes. Mix the flour and herbes de Provence together in a bowl and use to coat the meat. Add the meat to the pan and stir until sealed on all sides. Pour in the stock, the rest of the vegetables and the bay leaves. Cover and simmer for about 1½ hours until the meat is tender, adding water if it looks as if it's drying out. Remove and discard the bay leaves and serve with rice or mashed potato.

spinach with yoghurt

baby spinach leaves	900g
unsalted butter	25g
pumpkin seeds	3 tbsp
live natural yoghurt	150g

Wash the spinach and put into a saucepan with only the water clinging to it. Add the butter and pumpkin seeds. Cover and cook over a very low heat until the spinach is wilted, about 7 minutes. Drain, cool slightly and chop roughly. Stir in the yoghurt and serve.

grilled marinated fish

extra-virgin olive oil	4 tbsp
onion	1, small, very finely chopped
lime	juice of 1
mixed parsley, fennel fronds, dill, coriander and tarragon	4 tbsp, finely chopped
fish fillets, any variety	4
Cheddar cheese	2 tbsp, grated

Preheat the grill to high. Mix the oil, onion, lime juice and herbs together in a large, shallow dish. Add the fish and coat thoroughly in the marinade. Cover with clingfilm and refrigerate for at least 30 minutes.

Drain the fish, reserving the marinade. Place the fish on the grill pan and brush each side with the marinade. Cook for up to 5 minutes on each side, depending on the thickness of the fish. Sprinkle over the cheese and grill for a further 1 minute, until the cheese bubbles. Serve immediately.

mixed cabbage, leek and spring onions

This is the ultimate detoxing and health-boosting vegetable dish. Heart-protective, artery-friendly and anti-cancer nutrients abound. There's also lots of sulphur, so it's great for spotty skins.

walnut oil	3 tbsp
sesame oil	3 tbsp
Savoy cabbage	1, medium, finely shredded
leeks	3, cleaned and finely sliced
spring onions	6 plump, roughly chopped
carrots	2, grated
sesame seeds	2 tbsp
light soy or hoisin sauce	2 tbsp

Heat the oils in a large frying pan or a preheated wok. Add the vegetables and stir-fry until soft, stirring continuously, for about 10 minutes. Add the sesame seeds and soy or hoisin sauce and heat through for a further minute.

chicken jalfrezi

rapeseed oil	4 tbsp
cumin seeds	1 tsp
garlic	3 cloves, finely chopped
fresh root ginger	3cm, peeled and grated
turmeric	1 tsp
green Thai curry paste	2 level tbsp
chicken breasts	800g skinless, cut into thin strips along the grain
red chillies	2, deseeded and finely chopped
orange pepper	1, deseeded and cubed
tomatoes	1 x 220g can
coconut milk	125ml
coriander	2 tbsp chopped fresh
garam masala	2 tsp
cooked rice	to serve

Heat the oil in a large frying pan or preheated wok. Add the cumin seeds, garlic, ginger, turmeric, curry paste and 1 teaspoon of water. Add the chicken pieces, stir to coat in the spices and cook for 2 minutes. Add the chillies, pepper and tomatoes and simmer for 10 minutes. Pour in the coconut milk and add the coriander. Simmer for a further 5 minutes or until the chicken is tender. Add the garam masala and cook for 2 minutes. Serve with rice.

scrambled eggs with smoked mackerel

This sounds like a strange mixture, but it makes a delicious weekend brunch, breakfast or light supper. Smoked mackerel contains less salt than smoked salmon, has a fuller flavour and all the health benefits of oily fish.

smoked mackerel fillets	225g, flaked
single cream	3 tbsp
lemon	juice of ½
spring onions	4, large, finely chopped
butter	50g
eggs	6
parsley	2 tbsp finely chopped leaves
wholemeal toast	to serve

Mix the mackerel fillets with the cream, lemon juice and spring onions in a large bowl. Set aside. Heat the butter in a non-stick frying pan. Add the eggs and gently break up the yolks. Continue cooking, pushing the egg mixture in from the outside of the pan — you want the yolks and whites to stay slightly separate. When the eggs are beginning to set, add the mackerel mixture and cook until you have the consistency you prefer. Scatter with the parsley leaves and serve immediately with wholemeal toast.

roast lamb with rosemary

lamb	1 rack containing at least 8 chops
garlic	2 cloves, halved
olive oil	2 tbsp
herb salt	2 tsp
rosemary	2 large sprigs, cut into quarters

Preheat the oven to its highest setting. Rub the lamb with the cut side of the garlic halves, then with olive oil. Sprinkle over the herb salt. Make small incisions between each of the chops and insert the rosemary sprigs in the cuts. Place the lamb in a roasting tin and transfer to the preheated oven. Turn the oven down to 190°C/375°F/Gas 5 and leave to cook for 30 minutes.

bulgur with aubergine

bulgur wheat	225g
olive oil	8 tbsp
onion	1, large, finely chopped
aubergine	2, cubed
ground coriander	3 tsp
ground cumin	3 tsp
flaked almonds	150g
raisins	110g

Simmer the bulgur wheat in twice its volume of water until most of the water has been absorbed, about 10 minutes. Reserve until required. Meanwhile, heat the oil and fry the onion until golden. Add the aubergine and continue frying until both are crisp, adding more oil if necessary. Add the coriander and cumin and cook for 1 minute, stirring continuously. Reduce the heat, add the almonds and raisins and cook for 2 minutes or until the almonds are golden. Stir in the bulgur wheat, drained if necessary, and heat through for about 1 minute.

pasta noodles with broccoli

broccoli	350g small fresh florets – frozen won't work
egg linguini	400g
olive oil	4 tbsp
garlic	2 large cloves, finely chopped
anchovy paste	1 level tsp
red chilli	½, deseeded and very finely chopped
Parmesan cheese	4 tbsp, freshly grated

Blanch the broccoli florets in a saucepan of boiling water for 5 minutes. Remove from the water and reserve. Add the pasta to the water and cook according to the packet instructions. Meanwhile, heat the oil in a large frying pan and add the garlic, anchovy paste and chilli. Add the broccoli and continue cooking, stirring continuously, for 5 minutes. Drain the pasta. Pour the garlic, anchovy and chilli mixture over and serve immediately with the Parmesan cheese.

spicy chicken

chicken drumsticks	8
live natural yoghurt	200g
garlic	2 cloves, very finely chopped
paprika	2 tsp
ground coriander	1 tsp
lemon	juice of 1
extra-virgin olive oil	3 tbsp

Put the chicken in a wide, shallow dish. Mix the yoghurt, garlic, paprika, coriander, lemon juice and olive oil together in a bowl. Pour the mixture over the chicken, cover with clingfilm and leave to marinate in the fridge for 2 hours.

Preheat the grill and line a pan with foil. Remove the chicken from the dish, place on the grill pan and reserve the marinade. Brush the chicken with the marinade and cook under the preheated grill for about 20 minutes, turning frequently and basting with any extra marinade. Alternatively, cook on a barbecue.

salmon in a parcel

salmon fillets	4
extra-virgin olive oil	4 tbsp
tarragon	4 sprigs
parsley	4 tbsp chopped leaves
capers	2 tbsp, rinsed and chopped
lemon	4 slices

Preheat the oven to 200°C/400°F/Gas 6. Cut 4 pieces of kitchen foil large enough to make a parcel round the fish. Put the fish onto the foil and divide the olive oil, tarragon, parsley and capers between them. Top each with a slice of lemon. Fold the foil over and tuck in the ends. Place the parcels on baking sheets and cook in the preheated oven for 20 minutes.

pan-fried liver

rapeseed oil	4 tbsp
unsalted butter	50g
onion	1, large, finely chopped
unsmoked back bacon	4 thin rashers, cut in 2 lengthways
calves' liver	700g, thinly sliced
sherry	5 tbsp
parsley	4 tbsp finely chopped leaves

Liver is the organ that stores agricultural chemicals, so choose organic whenever you can. It's the richest source of vitamin A, contains the most easily absorbed iron and supplies lots of vitamins B12 and D. This is a quick, easy and healthy recipe – but not if you're pregnant as the huge amount of vitamin A could damage your baby.

Heat the oil and butter in a saucepan and sauté the onion and bacon until just turning gold. Remove with a slotted spoon and reserve. Add the liver to the pan and cook until just turning brown, about 1 minute on each side. Return the onion and bacon to the pan, pour in the sherry and heat until bubbling. Stir in the parsley and serve immediately.

braised chicken

rapeseed oil	4 tbsp
shallots	8, halved
smoked back bacon	4 rashers, snipped into 6 pieces each
chicken	1, weighing about 1.3 kilos
mushrooms	150g, sliced
white wine	100 ml
bouquet garni	1 sachet
bay leaves	2
small new potatoes	400g

Preheat the oven to 190°C/375°F/Gas 5. Heat the oil in a casserole dish large enough to hold the chicken. Sauté the shallots and bacon for 4 minutes, then remove from the dish and reserve. Add the chicken and brown on all sides. Return the onion and bacon to the dish, along with the mushrooms, wine, bouquet garni and bay leaves. Cover and cook in the preheated oven for 45 minutes. Add the potatoes and continue cooking for a further 30 minutes. Remove the bouquet garni and bay leaves before serving.

stuffed red peppers

red peppers	2, with flat bottoms, halved widthways and deseeded
extra-virgin olive oil	4 tbsp
onion	1, medium, finely chopped
garlic	2 cloves, finely chopped
pine kernels	2 tbsp
spinach	200g
Basmati rice	100g, cooked
Parmesan cheese	4 tbsp, freshly grated

Preheat the oven to 180°C/350°F/Gas 4. Put the peppers into a lightly greased baking tin. Heat the oil in a small saucepan and add the onion and garlic. Cook until the onion is soft. Add the pine kernels and continue cooking until the pine kernels are just golden.

Meanwhile, wash the spinach and put into a saucepan with just the water clinging to it. Cover and simmer gently until just wilted. Mix together the rice, garlic, onions, pine kernels and spinach. Pile the mixture into the 4 pepper halves, cover lightly with foil and cook in the preheated oven for 30 minutes. Remove the foil. Top with the Parmesan cheese and return to the oven for a further 10 minutes. Serve.

soups and salads

If you're taking the trouble and making the effort to detox, you're serious about your health. So you won't mind the extra work involved in making your own stock and good salad dressings – the rewards in terms of health-giving nutrients and absence of salt and unwanted chemicals far outweigh the effort.

very veggie stock

onions	2 – 1 peeled and quartered, 1 left whole
celery	3 large stalks, with their leaves
leek	1
parsnip	1
sage	1 large sprig
thyme	2 sprigs
bay leaves	6
parsley	2 generous handfuls
peppercorns	12, black, whole
water	2 litres

This basic recipe may seem as if it takes a long time and will leave you with far more stock that you need. But it's simple to make and healthier than any commercial stock or cube. If you don't need all of it, you can boil it down until it has reduced to half its volume, put it into the freezer – I often freeze it in ice-cube trays – then add it to an equal amount of boiling water and use as required.

Put all the ingredients into a large saucepan, cutting them to fit if necessary. Bring slowly to the boil and simmer for 40 minutes. Strain and use as required.

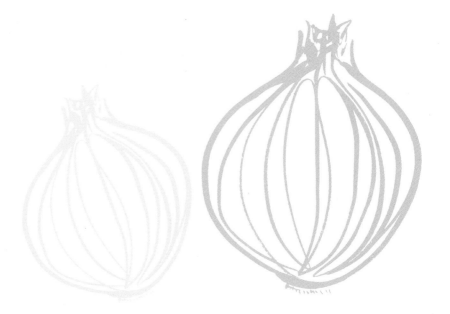

basic chicken stock

chicken	1 carcass – the remains of the Sunday roast will do, but it's better to ask a butcher to keep a carcass which has been stripped of its other useful meat
water	2 litres
spring onions	6, with the stems on
leek	1, large, trimmed and coarsely chopped
celery	2 large stalks, chopped
rosemary	1 large sprig
parsley	2 generous handfuls
sage	1 large sprig
thyme	2 large sprigs
bay leaves	3
white peppercorns	10

Put the chicken carcass into a large heavy-based saucepan and cover with the water. Bring to the boil and cook, uncovered, for 30 minutes. Add the rest of the ingredients, partially cover the pan and simmer for 40 minutes, adding more water if necessary. Strain and use as required.

my salad dressing

extra-virgin olive oil	300ml
white wine vinegar	100ml
Dijon mustard	1 tbsp
spring onions	2, very finely chopped
garlic	1 clove, very finely chopped
parsley	1 tsp freshly chopped leaves

Mix all the ingredients together in a bowl. Transfer to a screw-topped jar and shake well. Serve. This will keep for up to 2 weeks, unrefrigerated.

lettuce soup

Perfect as an evening snack as lettuce helps you sleep, and it's a great way to use up a glut of garden lettuces.

Heat the oil and sauté the onion gently for 2 minutes. Add the garlic and continue cooking for a futher 1 minute. Add the shredded lettuce and stir until wilted. Pour in the stock and tarragon and simmer for 5 minutes. Serve with spoonfuls of crème fraîche floating on top.

extra-virgin olive oil	4 tbsp
sweet Spanish onion	1, large, very finely chopped
garlic	2 cloves, very finely chopped
Little Gem lettuce	2 heads, shredded
very veggie stock (see recipe, page 97)	1 litre
tarragon	4 large sprigs, leaves freshly chopped
crème fraîche	100ml

vegetable soup

One bowl gives at least three portions of health-boosting vegetables.

Heat the oil and sauté the onions and garlic for 5 minutes. Add the carrots, leeks and courgettes and continue cooking for a further 5 minutes. Pour in the stock and tomato purée and simmer until the vegetables are soft. Add the parsley and peas and continue cooking for about 5 minutes.

onion	1, large, peeled and finely chopped
garlic	2 cloves, finely chopped
carrots	2, large, diced
leeks	3, trimmed, washed and sliced
courgettes	4, peeled and thinly sliced
very veggie stock (see recipe, page 97)	700ml
tomato purée	3 tbsp
parsley	1 large bunch, leaves finely chopped
peas	150g, fresh or frozen

chicken soup with barley

The ultimate healing soup, this is a one-pot meal providing protein, carbohydrates, vitamins, minerals and trace elements.

extra-virgin olive oil	4 tbsp
onion	1, large, finely chopped
carrot	1, large, finely sliced
leek	1, large, white part only, finely sliced
basic chicken stock (see recipe, page 98)	800 ml
pot barley	2 tbsp, washed
bay leaves	4
peppercorns	6, black
chicken carcass	1, skin removed
peas	50g, fresh or frozen
broad beans	50g, fresh or frozen

Heat the oil in a saucepan and sauté the onion, carrot and leek gently for 5 minutes. Add the stock, barley, bay leaves, peppercorns and chicken carcass. Cover and simmer for 2 hours, skimming away any scum that rises to the surface with a slotted spoon.

Remove the pan from the heat and leave to cool. Lift the chicken carcass out, remove any chicken meat from it and return the meat to the pan. Remove and discard the bay leaves. Add the peas and beans. Return the pan to the heat and simmer for 7 minutes.

borscht

This traditional Eastern European soup is excellent for general health, but especially valuable if you have anaemia, chronic fatigue or tired-all-the-time syndrome.

rapeseed oil	2 tbsp
onion	1, medium, peeled and finely sliced
garlic	2 cloves, finely chopped
fennel	1 large bulb, finely chopped
beetroot	400g, raw, peeled and finely sliced
carrot	1, large, peeled and sliced
very veggie stock (see recipe, page 97)	1 litre
thyme	1 large sprig
rosemary	1 large sprig
bay leaves	4
lemon	juice of 1
live natural yoghurt	150g, to serve

Heat the oil gently in a large saucepan and sauté the onion, garlic, fennel, beetroot and carrot for about 10 minutes. Pour in the stock and herbs and simmer for about 30 minutes until the vegetables are soft.

Remove and discard the herbs. Transfer the remaining ingredients to a food processor and whizz until smooth. Stir in the lemon juice. Serve with a swirl of yoghurt in each bowl.

thick bean and barley soup

The combination of cereal and legumes provides an abundance of protein, but the bonus comes from the plant hormones in the beans. Perfect for all menstrual problems and ideal for older women as it helps prevent bone loss – great for men, too.

pot barley	25g
very veggie stock (see recipe, page 97)	1 litre
carrots	3, medium, peeled and cubed
turnip	1, large, peeled and cubed
parsnip	1, medium, peeled and cubed
celery	2 stalks, with leaves, finely sliced
tomato purée	2 large tbsp
mixture of fresh chervil, parsley, oregano, marjoram and sage	4 large tbsp, finely chopped
borlotti, black-eye, red kidney, haricot, flageolet or other beans	1 x 250g can, well rinsed and drained
parsley	2 tbsp freshly chopped leaves, to garnish

Put the barley and stock in a large saucepan and simmer for about 40 minutes until the barley is soft. Add the vegetables, tomato purée and herbs. Bring back to the boil and simmer for a further 15 minutes. Add the beans and continue to simmer for another 15 minutes, until the beans are soft. Serve with the extra parsley scattered on top.

white soup

The best soup in the world to protect your heart.

ground almonds	175g
garlic	2 cloves, very finely chopped
white organic bread	2 thick slices, soaked in water and squeezed dry
extra-virgin olive oil	125ml
iced water	about 700ml
lemon juice	2 tbsp
seedless white grapes	20, halved

Put the almonds, garlic and bread into a food processor and whizz until smooth. Keeping the machine running, gradually add the olive oil until the mixture is the consistency of mayonnaise. Pour in the iced water until you have the texture of double cream. Stir in the lemon juice. Serve with the grapes floating on top.

onion soup

The traditional detox soup as well as being sometimes used to relieve bronchitis and other chest infections. What's more, it's a standard French cure for hangovers.

unsalted butter	50g
Spanish onions	2, peeled and sliced into rings
plain flour	1 tbsp
very veggie stock	900ml
(see recipe, page 97)	
thyme	4 large sprigs, leaves finely chopped
wholemeal bread	4 slices
Gruyère cheese	150g, grated

Preheat the grill and line a grill pan with foil. Heat the butter in a large saucepan. Add the onions and sauté until just turning golden. Add the flour, mix thoroughly and cook for 2 minutes. Pour in the stock and thyme and simmer for 10 minutes.

Meanwhile, toast the bread lightly and cut a circle out of each slice. Sprinkle the cheese on top and cook under the preheated grill until the cheese has melted. Serve the soup hot with the cheese-toasted bread floating on top.

oat and broccoli soup

This might sound like a cross between breakfast and lunch, but it tastes great. It is extremely cleansing as part of a detox regime and helps protect against heart disease and bowel cancer.

extra-virgin olive oil	2 tbsp
spring onions	6, chopped
broccoli	500g, cut into florets
porridge oats	60g
very veggie stock	500ml
(see recipe, page 97)	
semi-skimmed milk	500ml
nutmeg	½ tsp
single cream	2 tbsp
chives	10, snipped

Heat the olive oil in a large saucepan and sauté the spring onions gently until just soft. Add the broccoli and continue cooking, stirring continuously, for 2 minutes. Add the oats and stir for 1 minute. Mix together the stock and milk and add to the saucepan. Cover and simmer for 10 minutes. Add the nutmeg. Just before serving, stir in the cream and scatter the chives over the top.

carrot salad

carrots	4, medium, grated
flaked almonds	75g
raisins	50g
my salad dressing	100ml
(see recipe, page 98)	

Mix the first 3 ingredients together in a bowl. Stir in the salad dressing and blend thoroughly. Serve.

watercress salad

watercress	1 bunch or bag, rinsed (even if the packet says it's ready-washed) and all thick stems removed
red onion	1, large, very finely sliced
mint	4 large sprigs, leaves removed and roughly torn
lemon	juice of 1
olive oil	5 tbsp

No-one eats enough watercress. It's a good source of iron and vitamin C but, most importantly, it contains chemicals that protect specifically against lung cancer – vital for smokers.

Mix the watercress, onion slices and mint together in a bowl. Whisk the lemon juice and olive oil together and pour over the salad.

cucumber and strawberry salad

cucumbers	2, large, peeled and very finely sliced
rocket	3 sprigs, leaves finely torn
strawberries	10, large, hulled and cubed
balsamic vinegar	2 tbsp

Put the cucumber into a colander and sprinkle with salt. Leave for about 1 hour so all the water is drawn out. Rinse thoroughly and dry in a clean teatowel. Put the cucumber into a large bowl, add the rocket and strawberries and mix throughly. Sprinkle the balsamic vinegar over the top and serve.

avocado, tomato and mushroom salad

Bursting with protective antioxidants, especially vitamin E and lycopene, which help prevent some forms of cancer.

avocados	2, peeled, stoned and sliced lengthways
beef tomatoes	4, sliced widthways
close-cap mushrooms	110g, wiped and finely sliced
extra-virgin olive oil	about 5 tbsp
limes	juice of 2
black pepper	to serve

Arrange the avocado and tomato slices around the edge of four plates. Mix together the mushrooms, oil and lime juice and pile them in the centre of the plates. Serve with a generous twist of black pepper.

tsatsiki

As well as being good for your digestion, thanks to the mint and bacteria in the yoghurt, this also provides calcium for strong bones.

live natural yoghurt	250g
cucumber	1, medium, peeled, deseeded and finely grated
garlic	2 cloves, peeled and chopped
mint	5 sprigs, leaves removed, plus 4 sprigs to garnish

Put all of the ingredients except the mint sprigs into a blender. Whizz until smooth. Serve with the mint sprigs on top.

celery salad

celery	8 stalks
capers	4 tsp, rinsed
cottage cheese	200g
chives	10, finely snipped

Arrange the celery in 4 bowls. Bruise the capers with the back of a fork, then put them in a bowl, add the cottage cheese and mix thoroughly. Transfer the mixture to the 4 bowls and serve with the chives sprinkled on top.

fruit crudités with ricotta cheese dip

mixed fresh fruit	about 500g, peeled and cored if necessary, but leave apples, peaches, and pears unpeeled
ricotta cheese	2 x 100g tubs
mint	4 sprigs

Cut the fruit into bite-sized pieces and arrange around the edges of four large plates. Beat the cheese until smooth and pile in a mound in the middle of each plate. Serve with the mint sprigs garnishing the cheese.

tomato, red onion and beetroot salad

beef tomatoes	4, coarsely chopped
red onion	1, coarsely chopped
beetroot	3, medium, cooked (but not pickled) and diced
beansprouts	200g
my salad dressing (see recipe, page 98)	150ml
coriander	1 small bunch, leaves freshly chopped
mascarpone cheese	100g

Mix the first 4 ingredients together, tossing them well in a large bowl. Whisk the dressing, coriander and mascarpone cheese together in a separate bowl and drizzle it on top. Serve.

grapefruit, peach and fromage frais salad

pink grapefruit	2, peeled and cut into segments
peaches	4, stoned and cut into slices about the size of the grapefruit segments
spring onions	4, very finely sliced
fromage frais	200ml

Arrange the grapefruit and peach slices around the sides of a large serving plate. Put the spring onions and fromage frais into a blender and whizz until smooth. Drizzle the fromage frais dressing on top of the fruit and serve.

carrot and red cabbage salad

carrots	2, large, grated
red cabbage	½, finely shredded
apples	2, peeled and finely grated
red pepper	1, deseeded and finely cubed
plum tomatoes	4, quartered
radishes	10, quartered
celery	2 stalks, finely chopped
sunflower seeds	2 tbsp
extra-virgin olive oil	6 tbsp
lemon	juice of ½

This really is health on a plate as it contains enormous amounts of protective carotenoids and cleansing fibre. It also has a gentle diuretic action.

Mix the first 7 ingredients together in a bowl and blend thoroughly. Sprinkle the sunflower seeds on top. Whisk the olive oil and lemon juice together in a separate bowl, drizzle over the salad and serve.

index

picture credits

1 Gettyimages/Andrea Booher; 2-3 Digital Vision; 4-5 Digital Vision; 14-15 Gettyimages/Paul Stanier; 17 Gettyimages/VCL/Bronwyn Kidd; 24-25 Digital Vision; 27 ImageState; 28-9 Digital Vision; 31 Digital Vision; 35 Gettyimages/David Sacks; 36-7 Gettyimages/Garry Hunter; 43 Gettyimages/James Darrell; 44-5 Gettyimages/Marc Romanelli; 51 Diana Miller; 53 Digital Vision; 60-61 Digital Vision; 63 Digital Vision; 66 Digital Vision; 69 Gettyimages/Sarto-Lund; 72 Gettyimages/Peter Holst; 74-75 Gettyimages/Erlanson Productions; 76/77 Digital Vision

acknowledgements

Three years ago our farmer pal, Malc, asked if he could put four of his Highland cattle in our field for a couple of months. Happily for my wife, Sally, and me, these magnificent long-haired, long-horned and placid animals are still there. They've now been joined by Big Bill, a gorgeous Hereford bull, to whom this series of detox books is dedicated.

Bill is the epitome of health, energy and radiance. He's immensely strong, boundlessly active, and his wonderful mahogany-coloured coat has the feel and texture of the finest silk.

Whether you're reading Super Health Detox, Super Energy Detox or Super Radiance Detox, you could all learn from Bill. He lives in an organic field, where he eats what nature intended for him – natural grasses, wild flowers and herbs – which provide all his essential nutrients. If we all lived a little closer to nature, we'd all be healthier, more energetic and more radiant.

I have to thank Sally for her tireless efforts with the recipes, and everyone at Quadrille for the beautiful design of this book. Special thanks must go to Hilary Mandleberg for her understanding, insight and incredible patience.

Editorial Director: Jane O'Shea
Consultant Art Director: Françoise Dietrich
Art Editor: Rachel Gibson
Project Editor: Hilary Mandleberg
Production: Nancy Roberts

First published in 2003 by
Quadrille Publishing Limited
Alhambra House
27–31 Charing Cross Road
London WC2H 0LS

British Library Cataloguing-in-Publication Data
A catalogue record for this book is available from the British Library.

ISBN 1 844000 22 2
Printed in Spain